Career Paths in Human–Animal Interaction for Social and Behavioral Scientists

Career Paths in Human-Animal Interaction for Social and Behavioral Scientists is an essential text for students and professionals wanting to pursue a career in human-animal interaction (HAI). It is exclusively designed to navigate this field and provide information on the best education, training, and background one might need to incorporate HAI into a successful career.

Kogan and Erdman bring together a diverse range of insights from HAI social scientists who have secured or created their HAI job. The book highlights six categories of work settings: academia, private practice, corporations/for profit companies, non-profit organizations, government, and other positions, to show the growing number of opportunities to blend social science interests with the desire to incorporate HAI into their careers.

The book clearly outlines the career paths available to social science students and professionals, from careers connected to human services of psychology, therapy, social work, and journalism, to research or other scholarship.

Lori R. Kogan, **PhD,** is Professor of Clinical Sciences at Colorado State University, USA. She is the Chair of the Human-Animal Interaction section of the American Psychological Association and Editor of the *Human-Animal Interaction Bulletin*, an open-access, online publication supported by the American Psychological Association.

Phyllis Erdman, **PhD,** is a professor of counseling at Washington State University and is a licensed mental health counselor, and past chair of the Human-Animal Interaction section of Division 17 of the American Psychological Association. She has been working in the field of human-animal interaction for over ten years, including assessment of equine therapeutic interventions, pet grief, and documenting the need for emotional support animals.

Career Paths in Human-Animal Interaction for Social and Behavioral Scientists

Edited by Lori R. Kogan
and Phyllis Erdman

Routledge
Taylor & Francis Group

NEW YORK AND LONDON

First published 2021
by Routledge
52 Vanderbilt Avenue, New York, NY 10017

and by Routledge
2 Park Square, Milton Park, Abingdon, Oxon, OX14 4RN

Routledge is an imprint of the Taylor & Francis Group, an informa business

Library of Congress Cataloging-in-Publication Data
Names: Kogan, Lori, editor. | Erdman, Phyllis, 1949– editor.
Title: Career paths in human-animal interaction for social and
    behavioral scientists / edited by Lori R. Kogan and Phyllis Erdman.
Description: New York, NY : Routledge, 2021. | Includes
    bibliographical references and index.
Identifiers: LCCN 2020048067 (print) | LCCN 2020048068
    (ebook) | ISBN 9780367366148 (hbk) | ISBN 9780367366155
    (pbk) | ISBN 9780429347283 (ebk)
Subjects: LCSH: Social scientists—Vocational guidance. |
    Human-animal relationships.
Classification: LCC H62 .C3417 2021 (print) | LCC H62 (ebook) |
    DDC 304.2/7023—dc23
LC record available at https://lccn.loc.gov/2020048067
LC ebook record available at https://lccn.loc.gov/2020048068

ISBN: 978-0-367-36614-8 (hbk)
ISBN: 978-0-367-36615-5 (pbk)
ISBN: 978-0-429-34728-3 (ebk)

Typeset in Bembo
by Apex CoVantage, LLC

Contents

Introduction

Welcome, readers, to an entertaining and informative book on careers that include human-animal interaction (HAI). As you are undoubtedly aware, the field of HAI is relatively new—yet expanding rapidly. It is a field that cuts across disciplines, professions, and academic majors. This is a book created for the growing number of social science students (and professionals) who know they want to work with animals but "don't want to be a vet". We, the editors, have both been there. We, too, come from social science backgrounds (psychology) and knew we wanted our careers to include animals. We wondered (Kogan during graduate school and Erdman as an already established academician), how to create a career that filled this need. Unfortunately, when we were struggling with these issues, there were no resources to help guide us. Only with persistence, tenacity (and a fair amount of luck) did we manage to forge our own unique paths. Here we are, decades later, wondering how to make this experience easier for those of you currently facing similar challenges. Unfortunately, there is still a lack of information to answer the questions most frequently asked: "I want to work with animals; what type of education do I need? What path do I take? What should I major in? How do I get a job that incorporates HAI clinical work or research?"

Our intent in publishing this book is to help you with these questions—those of you wanting to work in the HAI field but uncertain what education, training, and background are needed and what future careers are possible. While traditionally, options for those wanting to pursue a career with animals were limited to veterinary medicine, fortunately, that is no longer the case. A growing number of people are just like you—drawn towards the social sciences (e.g., psychology, social work, human development and family studies, occupational therapy, etc.) but want a career that includes an HAI focus. Fortuitously, as the HAI field has grown, so too have the options for creating a successful career with opportunities to blend social science and HAI interests.

To help give you some direction and guidance, we invited a wide array of professionals—all with different careers and educational backgrounds—to share their stories with you. Firsthand, they tell how they became involved in HAI work. You will read about some who entered the field with an educational background specifically focused on HAI as well as many who have woven HAI work into their current work through various professional paths and opportunities. Our hope is that by reading these professionals' personal stories—how they became involved in HAI work, what their typical day looks like, and their career suggestions—your path becomes a bit easier.

Whether you are simply exploring options or seeking more specific answers, this book offers nuggets of wisdom from those who have successfully incorporated HAI into their careers, thereby filling the void of resources for those looking for guidance. Through reading their stories, you can glean insights into how you too can pursue a path that can lead to your dream job. We have found that HAI work adds a dimension of satisfaction and joy to our current professional careers, and we want you, as the reader, to find the same joy in your career. We are not implying that the road will always be easy or straightforward, but if you harness the passion you have for this work and use it as the motivation to take risks and think creatively, we believe you can achieve the kind of satisfying careers illustrated in the following chapters.

We sincerely thank each of our authors for reflecting on their work and their lives and sharing their personal challenges and successes. We also thank you, as the reader, for your interest in exploring ways to enrich and expand your career with the inclusion of human animal interaction work.

Lori R. Kogan, Ph.D.
Phyllis Erdman, Ph.D.

Part I
Academic—Traditional

1 From Biopsychology to Human Behavioural Work to HAI Research

One Academician's Path

Anne Barnfield

Anne Barnfield, DPhil, is an associate professor of psychology at Brescia University College. Her current research focuses on equine-assisted/ facilitated activities including beneficial influences of therapeutic riding (TR) for children with special needs, and applications of Equine-Assisted Therapy/Psychotherapy (EAT/EAP) for treatment of anxiety and post-traumatic stress disorder (PTSD) for military veterans and emergency services personnel.

The academic psychologist may be thought of as being on the more "scientific" side of psychology, and so on a straightforward career pathway. The course of an academician's research path, however, does not always take a straight line from A to B. One might start out in a specific field but then travel through a variety of areas within psychology across the course of a career, arriving at—perhaps—an unexpected destination!

The great thing about scientific research is that it is "finding out"— why things happen, what is going on, and how we can change behaviours. Research looks at "hows" and "whys" and understanding these so as to change things for the better—to be of use. Scientific method is objective and allows us to make reasoned decisions. Assumptions can be faulty; research helps us to arrive at factual conclusions.

It was the "finding out" aspect of scientific enquiry that first engaged me in my school years. Once I could make choices, I studied primarily scientific subjects. I continued my education, first using my scientific background to take a BSc degree—a joint degree, in psychology and biology. Here was my first turning point, branching off from "pure" science down a new, and different, pathway. Although it started as an interest, taken to fulfill a requirement, psychology became the focus of my studies. A course in biopsychology was another turning point—here was a perfect fit between the sciences of biology and chemistry and my new main interest, psychology. I went on to post-graduate studies, to a DPhil in experimental psychology. I moved further along what was becoming a winding path, allying biochemistry with behaviourism in behavioural analyses of drug effects on neurotransmitters.

My first post-doctoral position was as a research assistant in a neurochemistry laboratory. Although this seems like a purely psychobiology position, I brought behavioural analysis into the neurochemistry work being done in the department. Further post-doctoral positions were also in research laboratories, but now in universities. By this time, married to a Canadian, I had moved to Canada.

Changing place geographically led to changes in my research, something that often happens to academics. Once established in a full-time faculty position, I had to change my research focus. My path curved again, and I moved into more strictly behavioural work, with studies on spatial representations and development of spatial abilities, and some work on American Sign Language (ASL) and visuo-spatial abilities. As I moved on, I developed interest in the behavioural and cognitive effects of sport and exercise participation and began to study the effects of sport and physical activity, particularly child/youth participation.

At this point, a chance encounter led to another turn in the pathway. As a university faculty member, I was expected to supervise undergraduate research. I had become interested in horses and, with a student who shared my interests, planned a study on the effectiveness of TR, investigating TR's emotional and cognitive-behavioural effects. This branch of the pathway led me to a whole new area—the study of EAT/EAP's effects.

My current research is on the effectiveness of equine-assisted/facilitated interventions, particularly therapies/psychotherapies for mental health issues with a focus on the treatment of PTSD in military veterans and emergency services personnel. The findings so far are all positive: the participants have all been helped by EAT/EAP's and are enthusiastic about taking part in this type of therapy, more so than for other formats.

Being a university faculty member has challenges, but also benefits. Faculty are expected to engage in three main aspects of workload: teaching, research, and service (administration, committee work, etc.). Classes can be scheduled at different times and in different terms, meaning that one's schedule may completely change from semester to semester. For many faculty, most time spent outside of teaching time is dedicated to research and writing. Work often needs to be done at home, in evenings and on weekends; papers must be marked, research planned or written up, and so on. Academia is not a nine-to-five job!

An academic will, of course, study and work in a certain discipline; those interested in history work in that field, those interested in politics become political scientists. We choose those studies and work which are of most interest to us, but within specific areas situations often change. Whilst it is possible to plan out a research career in one, specific discipline, often the course is not clear—one has to go where work is available and take the positions offered. There are many graduates with master's and doctoral degrees, but fewer faculty positions; it may be difficult to find work directly in one's area of specialty. I would say, however, don't be afraid of not taking a straight-line route, but follow where the path leads. For myself, a long and winding pathway has led to an interesting career and a rewarding area of study: Human–Animal Interaction research.

2 A Twist in the Tale (or Is That Tail?)

How I Apply Health Psychology to the Human–Animal Bond

Anna Chur-Hansen

Anna Chur-Hansen is a professor who lives in Adelaide, South Australia. She holds a PhD in medical education, which she completed in the discipline of psychiatry in the School of Medicine at the University of Adelaide, and is a registered psychologist with an area of practice endorsement in health psychology from the Psychology Board of Australia.

———————

I am the first in my family to attend university. My parents were tradespeople—my father a small goods butcher, my mother a hairdresser. As a primary school student, I had a "calling"—I knew that I would one day work in a hospital. I had no role models and knew nothing about what that really meant, but I was strongly drawn to the health professions from a young age. In secondary school I volunteered every weekend at a nursing home where my career path was cemented. I started studying psychology at the University of Adelaide and worked at two nursing homes, every Saturday and Sunday morning for six years, to fund my studies.

In my early years we lived on a farm, and from birth I have always lived with domestic and other animals. At the time of writing I am the devoted fur-parent of a west Highland terrier, Clarence (Clarrie) Bruce Jones, and a cairn terrier, Ralph Albert (Bertie) Jones.

I am a professor at the University of Adelaide in the School of Psychology. I started my career as an academic in the School of Medicine, in psychiatry, based in the Royal Adelaide Hospital, where I taught medical students health psychology, psychological medicine and behavioural sciences. That was in 1987—I remained in psychiatry until the end of 2013, when I moved to psychology to become the Head of the School. I completed two terms as Head (six years), and currently I have returned to the role of teacher and researcher—in other words, a "regular" academic post.

I am endorsed as a health psychologist with the Psychology Board of Australia. As a health psychologist, I subscribe to the biopsychosocial model, and I conceptualise health as holistic and interrelated. I believe that our physical, mental, psychological, emotional, social, cultural, spiritual and community health all impact one another, and a person is best understood by considering all those component parts. Each week I consult at a general/family practice surgery and see up to four clients per week for various health-related presentations, drawing on that philosophical framework to inform my practice.

My research, teaching and clinical practice are all broadly around food and eating, sex and relationships, pain, and death and dying. My PhD was in medical education: I am very interested in the ways in which we train health professionals and how they, and their patients, experience interactions in health settings. Part of my work involves the study of the human-animal bond (HAB) from a biopsychosocial model. Not only do I apply HAB work in my clinical practice, I research the impact on people's mental and physical health, including people who work with animals, such as veterinarians and veterinary nurses.

I am privileged and blessed to have my career; I have the opportunity to study and research areas that can really make a difference in people's lives. I work with amazing students—from the incoming undergraduates to the honours, master's and PhD students I am fortunate to supervise. I get to meet, talk and collaborate with incredible colleagues in my own discipline and university, and also from all over South Australia, Australia and internationally.

There are of course challenges in working in the university sector and also in being a practising psychologist. Universities need to increase revenue and so academic staff must attract students and grant funding and publish high quality research in the best journals possible. Despite our best efforts, these can be somewhat uncontrollable outcome variables—competition is tough. As a psychologist, I find it important to look after myself; I regularly engage in peer supervision and take time for rest and reflection.

What Helped Me Succeed

Looking back on my trajectory, there are several factors that I think were central to helping me on my journey and which remain important. First, throughout my school years, I had a group of wonderful friends who kept me engaged and connected. One of those people remains my best friend; next year will be our 40th anniversary of meeting in a university tutorial class in Week 1 of Year 1. He still gives me career advice and wise words over dinner to this day.

Once I started working, I was very fortunate to meet several mentors who became instrumental to my career—I would encourage you to seek out people who can give you advice and encouragement, bounce around ideas with, and look for opportunities for you. Mentors were important in my volunteer work, not just in my paid roles. It can be an informal or formal arrangement—but the value of mentoring should not be underestimated. It will work best, I have found, if you and your mentor have synergy and enjoy one another's company.

Finally, for me, companion animals have been a source of social support and an inspiration for my research, teaching and practice. Additionally, they help me exercise, meet people both inside and outside academia, and connect online and in person with other like-minded individuals. I am quite sure that my quality of life would be much poorer without them.

3 Scientist-Practitioner Psychologist

Integrating the Human-Animal Interaction Into Practice

Jennifer Coleman

Jennifer Coleman, PhD, is an assistant professor in the Department of Psychiatry and Behavioral Sciences at Rush University Medical Center. Currently she works as a clinical psychologist for Rush's Road Home Program, a nonprofit that provides no-cost mental health services for veterans and their family members. In additional to clinical work, she enjoys teaching residents, supervising, and doing research.

I have loved animals since before I can remember. But it wasn't until I was applying for PhD programs that I realized I could specialize my education in the field of human-animal interactions (HAI). A professional in the field suggested I contact a leader in the field (Dr. Aubrey Fine) to discuss career options. He provided me with the best piece of advice I could have received, which I now pass down to anyone interested in this field. First, focus on a degree or license that will open doors to the career you want, then you can supplement your work with HAI education and training.

After earning a bachelor's degree in psychology and master's degree in mental health counseling, I knew I wanted a career that contained both research and clinical work. Thus, I applied to clinical and counseling psychology doctorate programs that had faculty who would support HAI research. I was lucky, as graduate programs are highly competitive and at the time focusing on HAI was novel, and I found a faculty advisor who wanted to begin researching HAI. I was also aware that Dr. Sandra Barker, Founder of the Center for Human-Animal Interaction, worked at the associated medical school down the road.

During my doctorate training I had two main objectives. The first was to specialize in trauma work, be competitive for a clinical internship, and eventually attain a career as a licensed clinical psychologist. The second was to engage in HAI research and educational activities. This always meant a constant balance between fulfilling my clinical requirements and obtaining HAI experience. For example, my master's thesis focused on service dogs whereas my doctorate dissertation focused on veterans with PTSD receiving group therapy. Thus, I focused on HAI research and had a clinically based research project to speak about on internship interviews.

This balance meant that I had to independently seek out HAI related experiences, such as mentoring undergraduates in HAI research, proposing a study on incarcerated individuals who worked with dogs, and working as a research assistant on a project examining animal-assisted therapy for children with autism spectrum disorders. I also initiated a project that involved consultation with various mentors to create a novel measure to assess attitudes towards dogs (Coleman et al., 2016).

Since graduating, I have obtained a position as a clinical psychologist and assistant professor at Rush University Medical Center's Road Home Program. Although my current job may not look exactly as I had envisioned, I believe I am on the path to creating my dream job. The majority of my time is spent conducting psychotherapy for veterans with post-traumatic stress disorder—work that I love. I am also engaged in clinical supervision, teaching medical residents and conducting research. A current research project I am leading involves assessing the benefits and challenges for veterans who have psychiatric service dogs. One aspect of my current position that can be challenging is protecting time for research since I work in a job that is grant funded for clinical work and I do not currently have grant funding to allow for protected time for HAI research.

My dream job would involve more HAI integrated work. Thus, the ongoing challenge I am faced with is how to further integrate this into my current job. I have had to be creative. For example, currently I serve as a journal reviewer for HAI related manuscripts, present at conferences on HAI topics, attend the International Society for Anthrozoology conference regularly, and serve on an American Psychological Association emotional support animal committee. Due to this work I have now become the subject matter expert at my job, and at times in my larger institution, on the topic of service animals. This has led to teaching grand rounds to the department and regularly lecturing to medical residents and psychology trainees on the topic. I have also considered obtaining a facility dog to bring to work to help reduce stress and burnout for clinicians bearing in mind the many logistical barriers and challenges that need to be considered before such an endeavor.

My connection to an academic medical center has also given me unique training experiences for which I am extremely grateful. For example, this year I am part of the OpEd Project Fellowship. It is a yearlong project to train underrepresented voices in speaking publicly through writing opinion pieces. Through this fellowship, one of the OpEd pieces I published ran in the *Chicago Sun-Times* related to the shortcomings of U.S. legislation regarding service animals and emotional support animals.

I have three recommendations for the next generation of HAI scholars and practitioners. The first is to connect. Network with others in the field, join HAI list serves, attend HAI conferences, subscribe to HAI journals, collaborate on research, find mentors, and support HAI organizations. The second is to promote evidence-based research to help grow the HAI field out of its infancy and into a more widely respected discipline based on well-conducted research. Last, be creative. There are a multitude of avenues you can take to create a career that involves HAI and for better or worse, there is no one right way to get to where you want to go.

Reference

Coleman, J. A., Green, B., Garthe, R. C., Worthington Jr, E. L., Barker, S., & Ingram, K. M. (2016). The Coleman dog attitude scale (C-DAS): Development, refinement, validation, and reliability. *Applied Animal Behaviour Science*, *176*, 77–86. doi:10.1016/j.applanim.2016.01.003

4   Dogs as Co-Researchers

Colleen Dell

Colleen Dell is a professor and Centennial Enhancement Chair in One Health and Wellness at the University of Saskatchewan in the Department of Sociology. She is a community-based researcher, and a large part of her team's research program involves working directly with therapy dogs, service dogs and companion animals. These projects include federal prisoners, university students, seniors, addictions treatment clients, war veterans and youth. She is also a co-founder of the PAWSitive Support Canine Assisted Learning program at Drumheller prison.

My interest in human animal interaction originated in 2013 during my sabbatical year as a sociology professor. I had studied mental health and addictions for the majority of my career, and I wanted to examine the field from a new standpoint. A colleague suggested that I identify a topic I love and would therefore enjoy studying, and the first thing I thought about was my canine companions! So I googled dogs and addiction and did not discover much. Now, seven years later, when I google these terms, much more peer reviewed research is available, including that of my team (see, for example, Effects of a Therapy Dog Program on the Wellbeing of Older Veterans Living in a Long Term Care Residence in *Human-Animal Interaction Bulletin*, 2018).

As a sociologist, my academic and applied approaches to addictions and mental health emphasize social justice. There is inherent similarity between human and animal social justice issues, but I was not exposed to this during my sociology degrees in Canada. I did not recognize, for example, that there is a linkage between animal cruelty and domestic violence. My sociological training nonetheless did prepare me for my current focus on human animal interaction in other ways, and in particular, my attention to community-based research and Indigenous health, both of which have informed my current work. The former emphasizes the need to equally account for multiple perspectives in the research process, and the latter includes animals and the environment as integral to understanding human wellness.

When I decided to focus on human animal interaction for my academic sabbatical, I signed up for a dog psychology course at Extreme K-9 in Illinois, USA. My past attention to Indigenous health and its recognition of animals and nature encouraged me to think outside my Western worldview. As a community-based researcher, I knew that if I was to work and study with dogs on my team then I needed to better understand my canine partners and ensure their lived experience is represented in all aspects of my work and to the best of my ability. I was challenged to use my sociological imagination and account for animals in social life at both the individual and institutional levels.

What I Do During an Average Day

There is no average day for me, and that is what I enjoy most about my job as an academic generally, and even more so working with dogs! Unique to my position is that I get to work with the three dogs I live with and consider members of my family. I am involved in various applied research projects with therapy dogs Kisbey, Anna-Belle and E-Jay, and each is a unique experience. For example, I work with therapy dog Anna-Belle at a forensic center with incarcerated patients in a research project evaluating the efficacy of animal assisted therapy alongside counsellors and patients. My team does several media releases a year to share our research findings and raise awareness about animal assisted interventions. Frequently, therapy dog Kisbey, who is now semi-retired, joins me in doing presentations and to represent the canine side of our work. She is also frequently featured in a daily post on a Facebook site I have been maintaining since 2013 (visit Anna Belle & Subie's Adventures). I also work on a daily basis with a service dog in training, E-Jay, as part of a national study I lead about the role of service dogs in the lives of veterans diagnosed with PTSD and struggling with problematic substance use. I have also responded to community crises with my therapy dogs and contributed to the policy discussions that ensued about their inclusion. These daily experiences inform every aspect of my research and practice, from the research questions I ask to consideration of the dogs' welfare when working.

Challenges Associated With My Job

The challenges I have as an academic are amplified when working with the dogs as a part of my team. As a community-focused institution, I am fortunate that my university is supportive of 'non-traditional' academic contributions. For example, I have two peer-reviewed publications with my therapy dog Anna-Belle as a co-author to recognize her experience (at least through my lens) (see, Questioning "Fluffy": A Dog's Eye View of Animal-Assisted Interventions (AAI) in the Treatment of Substance Misuse, in *Substance Use & Misuse*, 2015 & "She Makes Me Feel Comfortable": Understanding the Impacts of Animal Assisted Therapy at a Methadone Clinic, in *Canadian Journal of Aboriginal HIV/AIDS Community-Based Research*, 2019). I don't imagine this would be true of all academic institutions. By far, however, the greatest challenge with my job has been the passing of my research partner, service and therapy dog, Subie. I was not prepared for the public nature of his passing because of his integrated role in my academic and local community. However, on the positive side, this experience has given me intimate insight into the human animal bond and thus the humans I do research by, for and in partnership with.

Is This Type of Job for You and What Are Desirable Characteristics for Success?

I am frequently asked how someone can get into the human animal interaction field because they too would like to bring their dog to work. The question I respond with is, does your dog want to go to work with you? Placing the animal, and what little we truly know about them, at the center of our research and practice is the most desirable characteristic to work in this field. The Extreme K-9 dog psychology course I graduated from opened with the question 'Will you still love me when you understand who I really am?' I did not recognize then, but I do now, that the dogs I research alongside are co-researchers in every traditional sense of the word, and more. Understanding who they really are, to the best of our human ability, is necessary so we do not perpetuate biases and discrimination based on speciesism. To achieve this, we need to commit to asking questions that are not being asked, being open to searching for what is invisible and unspoken, and to working outside our disciplines. In short, working in the human animal interaction field as an applied academic researcher requires intense humility.

5 From an Animal Shelter Towards a Professorship in Anthrozoology

An Unusual Career Path

Marie-Jose Enders-Slegers

Marie-Jose Enders-Slegers, PhD, is a professor in anthrozoology at the Faculty of Psychology, Open University Heerlen, the Netherlands. She is a clinical and health psychologist, and her field of interest is the human-animal bond and animal-assisted interventions in health care and education. She is currently serving as the President of IAHAIO—International Association of Human Animal Interaction Organizations.

It never ever crossed my mind that I would eventually have a career as a professor in anthrozoology—yet, at 68 years of age, that is exactly what happened. I'm still very grateful for this opportunity, and thankful to the open mind of the dean and rector of the Open University in the Netherlands and the organization AAIZOO (Animal Assisted Interventions in Care, Research and Education) that created an endowed chair position.

Born in 1945, and growing up in a family with six children, it was not at all natural or expected that I would go to a gymnasium (preparatory high school). Yet, that is what I wanted to do. I was the oldest, a girl, and destined to help my mother in the household. It would be my two brothers who would have the chance to study. In those days, where I am from, men were expected to achieve outside the home, while women were expected to become mothers and spouses—so advanced education for women was not necessary. And yes, after attending a school (lyceum) for girls, I learned how to run a household and took some beginning level jobs (as a dental assistant, an assistant in a language laboratory, a secretary in a psychiatric hospital and a secretary of the Director in a general hospital). I worked at these jobs until I met my husband, a medical doctor, and married at the age of 24. My life then was all about marriage, raising my three children and assisting my husband in his office, day and night. My family also consisted of two dogs, three cats, two horses and chickens. We had a very busy social life, yet, for me, my life was not satisfying; I was not happy with the limited roles I was asked to play. I wanted to be more than the wife of, the mother of, the assistant of—I wanted to be myself.

When I was 40 I changed my life. I passed exams to be admitted to a university and since there was a huge problem of stray dogs in my village, I founded a shelter for abandoned animals. I enjoyed studying clinical and health psychology and excelled, although my life at that time was extremely challenging as I worked to keep all the different balls in the air: taking care of the family, helping in the medical practice of my husband, fulfilling social duties, working in the shelter as chair and as volunteer, and studying. Yet, I was drawn to do even more. Being in the shelter and experiencing the sad animals and the grief and sorrow of the elderly people who had to abandon these animals broke my heart. It drove me to get involved in the Regional Animal Protection Movement—first by becoming a board member and later president of the National Animal Protection Movement—working to implement changes in animal shelters and in the way we treat animals.

I managed to get my drs. (master's) degree in 1990 and was immediately appointed at the University of Utrecht. I had to promise that I would continue towards a PhD, however, in my own time, alongside my work as assistant professor. This I did, and I chose to research the influence of dogs and cats on the quality of life of the elderly. Having experienced in the shelter how the forced abandonment of pets impacted the elderly who had to move to a home for the elderly or a nursing home, drove my desire to investigate the meaning of pets for the elderly and try to bring about some change. That was quite a challenge. The topic I wanted to study was not taken seriously. Only one professor, Dr. M. van Son, my supervisor, believed in the value of my research. My colleagues, at times, spoke disparaging about my research, 'Studying the human-animal bond, is that science?'

During the ten years that I worked on my thesis (in my free time) I attended nearly all conferences of ISAZ (International Society of Anthrozoology), became a board member of the American Humane Association (two terms) and participated in IAHAIO (International Association of Human Animal Interaction Organizations) Conferences. All of these experiences broadened my vision about what was happening in the world in the field of human-animal interactions/bond (HAI/B). It was great to meet and work with so many bright people, passionate about our field, all of whom were working hard to establish a solid body of HAI/B knowledge. One key lesson I learned was that only by transparency, sharing and working together (researchers and practitioners) can we enhance and strengthen the field, a message I express as the current president of IAHAIO.

In addition, I founded organizations in the Netherlands to professionalize the field, to address the link between animal abuse and domestic violence, and help support the development of researchers and professionals in the field. In 2013 I started to work as a professor at the Open University, Faculty Psychology, and I currently supervise 12 PhD students—all working in the marvelous field of anthrozoology.

This career path has been (and still is) a life of hard work and long days (often 7am to 9pm), however, it brings me so much pleasure and satisfaction. It is a great reward to witness, at the end of my career, the success of my endeavors and see my research taken seriously—thereby fostering positive changes for the well-being of both people and animals.

6 There Is a Shelter Dog in My College Classroom

Shlomit Flaisher-Grinberg

Shlomit Flaisher-Grinberg, PhD, is an assistant professor of psychology and co-coordinator of the interdisciplinary neuroscience minor at Saint Francis University in Loretto, Pennsylvania. She teaches classes including Canine Learning & Behavior and Animal Minds and specializes in experiential learning. She maintains an active research lab where she investigates the effects of the human-animal bond on health and well-being.

I was trained as a neuropsychologist. The field of neuropsychology aims to study the interaction between the brain, nervous system, cognition, and behavior. After many years in research, I decided to combine my love of science with my love of teaching and accepted a position as a tenure-track assistant professor of psychology. Although some of the courses that I was charged to teach were within my field of expertise (e.g., biological psychology, psychopharmacology), other courses required a lot of preparation. One of them was "Learning", a class which Focuses on the theoretical basis of human learning. The field encompasses complex theories, principles and terminology (e.g., classical and operant conditioning), but it also offers practical tools that are relevant to many situations, conditions, and species. Specifically, the processes that govern human learning are the same ones that affect animal learning.

I thus designed lab-sessions and research-projects which required my students to apply their learning to the training of live rats. Although rats have a bad reputation, they are in fact clean, sociable, and smart. There is a great joy in the ability to teach rats to ride tiny scooters, push miniature shopping-carts, bowl, complete custom-built agility courses, or paint with their paws. There is also a benefit to the learning outcomes, as the acquired knowledge can be implemented towards the work with other animals (e.g., zoos/wildlife-rehabilitation centers), or with human patients (e.g., developmental disorders, addiction, etc.). Moreover, as my students learned to care for the health and well-being of the rats (providing a clean and stress-free environment, food, water, and enrichment), they also learned to respect their capabilities, and follow the ethical guidelines that pertain to the work with live animals. In fact, many of my students grew to love their rats, and several students chose to adopt them at the end of the semester.

A year later, I became intrigued with another teaching opportunity: shelter dogs. One of the factors which may facilitate or hinder the successful adoption of a dog from a shelter includes its behavioral repertoire. Specifically, a dog which displays fearful, aggressive, destructive, over-excitable, or disobedient behaviors may spend a long time at the shelter or may not find its forever home. While shelters are full of dedicated staff and volunteers, their ability to offer behavioral rehabilitation is subjected to time and funding constrains. I thought, what if we could use the knowledge and practices offered by the field of "Learning", and the resources that are inherent to higher education institutions to make a difference in the lives of shelter dogs, one dog at the time?

I, therefore, designed a new undergraduate psychology curricular item, titled the "Canine Learning and Behavior" course. I wanted my students to work with shelter dogs which have been abandoned, neglected, and abused (and as a result, display an array of health and behavioral issues), with the goal of providing these dogs with training and behavioral rehabilitation to improve the likelihood of their successful adoption. In order to accomplish this goal, I established a partnership with a local shelter and recruited an experienced, certified dog trainer as my adjunct instructor. I then secured dog-approved, on-campus housing and classrooms, notified campus police about the presence of dogs on the campus property, and generated dog-handling and training protocols which were reviewed and approved by our "Institutional Animal Care and Use Committee". Finally, I designed lectures and lab-based sessions which targeted the extinction of maladaptive behaviors, and training for obedience, agility, and socialization.

Thus far, I have taught the course four times. Many of the dogs selected for the course displayed behavioral and health-related issues, were older, belonged to the pit bull breed, and spent over a year at the shelter. All were successfully adopted at the end of the semester. In fact, we celebrate the end of each semester with a "Puppy-Graduation Ceremony", which includes paw-shakes, the handout of ACK-CGC certificates, Saint Francis University "Diploma", collar-tags, and a cake (liver and peanut butter for dogs, chocolate and vanilla for humans).

The teaching of animal-integrated courses within an academic institution requires a great deal of preparation and flexibility. Securing a budget (animal food), setting (animal-approved classrooms/housing), community partners (animal shelters), and protocols (planning for unexpected events) calls for the generation of collaborative partnerships with multiple academic offices. It also requires the recruitment of knowledgeable adjunct instructors (my academic education did not prepare me to train dogs) and the enrollment of enthusiastic, dedicated, and responsible students.

Taking a larger perspective on the topic, my role as faculty in higher education has both advantages and disadvantages. This is a demanding line of work. From class construction, teaching, and grading, to committee service, scholarship, and publication, it is hard to maintain a life-work balance, and I always take work home with me. On the other hand, the opportunity for life-long learning is irreplaceable, and the ability to work with accomplished colleagues, talented students, and enthusiastic community partners is unmatched. Moreover, the incorporation of animals into my classroom, as a part of the psychology curriculum, has dramatically enhanced my work satisfaction. My students perceive the class as instrumental for their personal and professional development; faculty, staff, administrators, and students enjoy the presence of dogs on campus; and I find myself smiling every day on my way to work. Given this positive experience, I was able to integrate animal visits into additional courses (e.g., roosters, bunnies, ferrets, and cats in my "Animal Minds" class), and I am currently working on the generation of a campus-based "shelter-dogs theme-house". This "living-learning" environment will enable students to foster and train shelter dogs throughout the entire academic year, while promoting academic excellence, meaningful residential experience, and community engagement. Potentially, it may serve as a local educational center to our campus and surrounding community, sharing knowledge in regard to dog training and working to eliminate animal neglect, cruelty, and abuse.

7 Human-Animal Interaction in Clinical Psychology

Teaching, Research, and Practice

Angela K. Fournier

Angela K. Fournier, PhD, is a licensed psychologist in Minnesota. She is certified to provide equine-assisted psychotherapy (EAP) in the Eagala model. She is also the Director of the Human-Animal Interaction Laboratory where she studies the psychological processes and outcomes of human-animal interaction, focusing on development of theory and validated measures.

I am a professor of psychology and licensed psychologist who specializes in human-animal interaction (HAI). Like many of the professionals in this book, my career in HAI is quite broad and includes multiple roles. These roles can be categorized broadly as teaching, research, and clinical practice.

Teaching, Research, and Practice

I am a professor in the Department of Psychology at Bemidji State University, a mid-size liberal arts university in northern Minnesota, USA. My main role is to teach undergraduate courses in psychology. In addition to core courses in the major, I teach a special topics course on the psychology of HAI. The most rewarding aspect of teaching is witnessing students grow as they move through their studies and prepare for the next steps in their career. As the Director of the Human-Animal Interaction Laboratory, within the Department of Psychology, I work with students and community collaborators to conduct research in HAI. Our research focuses on the development of validated measures and theoretical frameworks to explain the processes and outcomes of animal-assisted interventions. My favorite thing about research is that it is an adventure. There are highs and lows, it can be fast-paced, and the outcomes can be surprising. Currently, I spend just a few hours a week providing clinical services. This includes providing individual counseling to college students at our university counseling center and co-facilitating EAP sessions at a local private practice.

An Average Day

During the semester, I am on campus four days per week, for about eight hours per day. My hours depend on my teaching schedule but are usually 9am–5pm. On a typical day, I teach a couple of classes, meet with students for help with coursework or advising, participate in committee meetings, and prepare the next day's classes (e.g., create lectures, create and grade assignments). I teach both on campus and online. I work off campus one day per week, engaging in research, program development, or clinical practice of EAP. My schedule varies from day-to-day; it is never boring.

Background

My interest in anthrozoology dates back to growing up in rural North Dakota surrounded by animals. Although I understood the power of animals for human health and well-being on a personal level, I did not initially seek a career in the field. As a first-generation college student, I began my undergraduate work in the social and natural sciences. I eventually set my sights on a career in clinical psychology, pursuing a PhD at Virginia Tech. Inspired by the animals in my life and supported by my mentors, I began applying psychology to understand interactions between humans and animals. Once I completed my education, I began working as a faculty member in psychology. After several years of teaching and conducting research, I was introduced to EAP. I became certified as a mental health specialist through Eagala, the Equine Assisted Growth and Learning Association. I now co-facilitate EAP sessions, conduct research on EAP process and outcome, and serve on the Eagala research committee.

Freedom and Flexibility: Benefits and Challenges

Working in academia allows for a great deal of freedom and flexibility, which can be both a blessing and a curse. I am able to select my teaching schedule and office hours and can work from home when I don't have something scheduled on campus. However, because it is so flexible there aren't built-in boundaries to ensure a healthy balance between work and personal life. There is a lot of work to do—prepare the next class, answer emails, serve a committee or a community organization—and the work is portable. So there is always work that I *could* bring home. With mentoring, I learned the necessity of setting my own boundaries, which means deciding when to work and when to rest, as well as which work to take on.

Changes Based on Season/Time of Year

Faculty workload varies by time of year, which is one of the things I like best about the job. My faculty position is a nine-month contract, so I typically work full-time from mid-August until mid-May. That time frame is broken down into two semesters—fall and spring—separated by several weeks for winter break. I am not scheduled to work in the summer but can teach classes if I choose, depending on student need. For me, summer is a time to relax and refresh, as well as catch up on non-teaching activities like research, writing, and practicing EAP. In addition to the break in the winter and the long break in the summer, I enjoy the semester schedule—classes begin, run for 15 weeks, and then end. This cycle provides closure at the end of a semester and opportunity for revision and improvement when teaching a class more than once.

In summary, my HAI work involves teaching courses in the psychology of human-animal relationships, conducting research on how animals impact us, and incorporating animals in clinical practice. My path was to complete a doctorate degree in clinical psychology, become licensed and begin a program of research, and then get certified to incorporate animals in psychotherapy and learning. A full-time faculty position allows me to do all of these things I love, creating a sense of academic adventure.

8 An Entangled Path

Human Animal Interaction and Social Work

Cassandra Hanrahan

Cassandra Hanrahan is an associate professor and undergraduate program coordinator at Dalhousie University School of Social Work in Nova Scotia, Canada. Her research on human animal interactions in social work focuses on the reconceptualization of the purpose and practice of social work today. As part of this work, she raises awareness of anthropocentrism and a much needed critique of the human privilege that fortifies humanism in social work.

Inspiration/Revelation

My teaching and research about human animal interaction (HAI) in social work are inspired by an affinity with the more-than-human world. I grew up on the Atlantic coast of Canada, in a small town nestled in the Tantramar Marshes, or Tintamarre, as Acadians called it, referencing the racket made by raucous birds who feed there, and the rushing sound of tidal waters filling the Chignecto Bay. In Indigenous oral tradition, the Tantramar was alluded to as a meeting place through which Mi'kmaq bands moved seasonally from sea coast to inland forest (Mount Allison University Archives). As a child, this expansive tidal saltmarsh, hugging the Bay of Fundy, steeped in cattails and tadpoles, wild flowers, bogs, sandpipers, and dykes, was sacred in its natural splendour.

It seemed to me to be neither land nor sea, all sky and wind, an open pulsing heart. That place—for it was a *meeting* ground—gave me my first sense of *becoming*, as it transformed, without contradiction, the spaces in-between people, other animals, and the more-than-human world. The diversity of all that was consoled me. I was inspired, even frightened, by the raptors, eagles, and marsh hawks whom I thought might someday swoop down and pluck me up like a muskrat or rodent out of the melee of tall field grasses of every colour imaginable. A geographical borderland, a space within, the Tintamarre was for me a strength and a liability. In my bi-lingual, bi-cultural family there was much slippage among positions that define themselves one against another: civilized/uncivilized, culture/nature, human/animal; male/

female. I was never wholly one or the other, but rather entangled amidst the spaces between earth and water, land and sky, existence and culture, where people and other animals are "*a part* of the world rather than *in* the world" (Bozalek, 2016, p. 83). In those spaces-cum-places, different ways of being with different beings were created that have informed my living ever since.

I tell you this story of attunement—being and becoming aware, responsive—because it is this form of "agential realism" (Barad, 2007), more than anything, that informs my understanding of the social work values of justice, integrity, and equity (Hanrahan, 2011). Attunement with the more-than-human world, beyond the self, beyond species, *becomes* a moment of peaceful trans-species co-existence, and requisite methodological way towards sustainable individual and public health and well-being. Radical relationality (Braidotti, 2018) strengthens justice work by expanding its scope, facilitating not only an analysis of dominant discourse, its intrinsic 'othering' practices, and the way power is exercised in particular as privilege and oppression, but importantly, a critique of the profession's foundations—humanism and "anthroprivilege"; that is, "the ways in which humans take our species positionality for granted" (Springer, 2021, advance copy, p. 3). This re-perspectivizing of anthropocentric self-reflexivity (predominant methodological tool of critical practice) presents a new ethics of relationality that decenters humans, allowing the forces of empathy, care, solidarity and sympathy "to be transferred across positions of 'difference or alterity,' rather than necessitating 'sameness' for ethical behavior" (Fielder, 2013, pp. 501–502, citing Oliver, 2009, p. 21).

Challenges/Actions/Reckoning

When I began my research on HAI in social work just over ten years ago, a book about HAI career paths was implausible. Since, HAI studies has significantly impacted not only the social and behavioral sciences but much of the academia. The opportunity to share a little about my path as a Canadian social scientist within this context is momentous, in part because of the silence of Canadian social work concerning the extraordinary implications of HAI research for justice work, and in part because of the moral injury sustained due to my commitments to those ideas.

The primary requirement for a Canadian university faculty position is a doctorate degree (PhD). For an academic appointment in one of Canada's accredited social work programs, a master of social work (MSW) is required if one's PhD is in another field. A substantive area of expertise is another requisite. For those interested in HAI in social work and related topics like One Health (Hanrahan, 2015) and the environment, these are developed as complementary sub-specialties. In other words, one must establish themselves as a social work academic first, an HAI proponent second; often independently and resourcefully through a combination of campaigning and resilience. Canadian social scientists affiliated with social work and interested in HAI are few but growing and dispersed across the country. HAI opportunities must be actively sought and fostered nationally and internationally.

As a transdisciplinary field, HAI studies are rigorous. Developing and advocating for HAI in social work involves engaging several bodies of knowledge critically and creatively. The study of HAI emboldens the social work curriculum and holds the capacity to transform and sustain the profession by making it relevant to multiple contemporary realities including climate crisis and zoonotic infectious diseases. Raising awareness, whether about mutually beneficial animal assisted interventions or complex philosophical questions about animal beings and minds, sometimes elicits derision. Resisting human supremacy manifest, albeit differentially, across cultures, race and ethnicities, and its attendant human privilege, which "is the height of human hubris, precisely because it is the foundational moment of the construction of the 'self', and thus the bedrock upon which all forms of othering are structured" (Springer, 2021, p. 6), paradoxically can be subject to suspicion regarding one's commitment to social work and to people. Educational counter measures include finding kindred spirits and collaborators, developing an HAI study/reading group, teaching HAI independent studies and electives, guest lecturing, incorporating HAI themes into core courses, and presenting/publishing across disciplines and professions.

HAI in social work is an enormously rich field that can foster "radical relationality, non-unitary identities and multiple allegiances" (Braidotti, 2013, p. 144); new ways of being for a new "global polity" (Bauman, 2018). My HAI career path has as its guiding focus a paradigm shift. As one of the few professions wholly dedicated to social justice, it is time for social workers and critical social scientists alike to become, what I have called elsewhere, "animal-informed" (Hanrahan & Chalmers, 2020), and to break the cognitive dissonance that essentially limits the transformative potential of contemporary critical, otherwise counter practice and narratives.

References

Barad, K. (2007). *Meeting the universe halfway: Quantum physics and entanglement of matter and meaning.* London: Duke University Press.

Bauman, W. A. (2018). Religion, science, and nature: Doing without human exceptionalism. *Religious Studies Review, 44*(4), 383–388.

Bozalek, V. (2016). The political ethics of care and feminist posthuman ethics: Contributions to social work. In R. Hugman & J. Carter (Eds.), *Rethinking values and ethics in social work* (pp. 80–97). London: Palgrave Macmillan.

Braidotti, R. (2013). *The posthuman.* London: Polity.

Braidotti, R. (2018). A theoretical framework for the critical post humanities. *Theory, Culture, & Society,* 1–31. doi:10.1177/0263276418771486

Fielder, B. N. (2013). Animal humanism: Race, species, and affective kinship in Nineteenth century abolitionism. *American Quarterly, 65*(3), 487–514. doi:10.1353/aq.2013.0047

Hanrahan, C. (2011). Challenging anthropocentricism in social work through ethics and spirituality: Lessons from studies in human-animal bonds. *Journal of Religion and Spirituality in Social Work: Social Thought, Special Edition, 30*(3), 272–293. doi.org/10.1080/15426432.2011.587387

Hanrahan, C. (2015). Integrative health thinking and the new *one health* concept: All for 'one' or 'one' for all? In T. Ryan (Ed.), *Animals in social work: Why and how they matter.* London: Palgrave Macmillan.

Hanrahan, C., & Chalmers, D. (2020). Animal-informed social work: A more-than-critical practice. In C. Brown & J. MacDonald (Eds.), *Critical clinical social work: Counter storying for social justice* (pp. 195–223). Toronto: Canadian Scholar's Press.

Mount Allison University Archives. *First people and the marsh, marshlands: Records of life on the Tantramar.* Retrieved February 27, 2020. www.mta.ca/marshland/topic2_first people/firstpeople.htm

Oliver, K. (2009). *Animal lessons: How they teach us to be human.* New York: Columbia University Press.

Springer, S. (2021). Check your anthroprivilege! Can we make space for intersectionality when cognitive dissonance prevails? In P. Hodge, A. McGregor, Y. Narayanan, S. Springer, O. Veron, & R. White (Eds.), *Vegan geographies.* Retrieved July 15, 2020. www.researchgate.net/publication/336374517

9 Solidarity and Scholarship

Thriving as an HAI Academic

Rachel Caroline Hogg

Rachel Caroline Hogg is a psychology academic at Charles Sturt University, Australia, with a PhD in equestrian psychology. She researches human-animal interaction, with a special interest in horse-human relationships and animal-assisted therapies. She is particularly concerned with the implications of animal labor in sporting, therapeutic, and educational contexts, and the theoretical intersections between critical psychology, ecopsychology, gender studies, and animal lives.

Animals have been at the centre of my life as far back as my memory extends, a child growing up on a wheat and sheep farm in Australia. Psychology came later, an emergent pathway into the push and pull of human life. The idea that animal lives were insignificant in contrast to human lives was never explicitly expressed to me; in contrast, (pet) animals were treasured family members and our sheep were critical to the farming business. Similarly, animals have in some ways been consequential to psychology, but in both the personal and the professional, context is critical. My mother cared for our horses in the same way she cared for us, her children, and it was through her actions that I began to understand that elevating animals was not a cognitive error, but an invitation into what would become the most critical part of my interest in human-animal studies: the juncture between human and animal.

As an undergraduate psychology student in the late-2000s, I moved within an intellectual context that I did not fully understand, but that nonetheless informed what I thought was possible. Psychology has an ambiguous history with the personal. The 'personal' is, as second-wave feminism told us, 'political', and psychology has historically distanced itself from anything seen as compromising the objective, apolitical, experiential framework that underscores scientific legitimacy. In particular, psychology has disavowed art, subjectivity, emotion, the body, and 'the animal other'; though slowly the tides are turning. I had not considered the idea that my own interest in animals might shape my career, despite the fundamentally relatable nature of psychology as a discipline. I was never actively discouraged from thinking about things that I cared about, but underpinning my tertiary education was the unspoken need to maintain emotional distance from my work endeavours, even as a student.

Years later, sitting in my future honours supervisor's office in the final year of my undergraduate degree, I was asked the predictable, yet disarming question, "What would you like to research?" I was certain about my interests, but had not anticipated such freedom, aware that many universities expected students to fit into neatly demarcated research programs. My supervisor, by his own account, was far from an equine enthusiast or human-animal researcher, but offered to supervise my research on anxiety in equestrian athletes, and so began a formative year of work. Only in hindsight was I able to recognise the significance of this period. I was not drawn towards clinical psychology, but I was enthralled by research and the possibilities it offered. Consequently, I embarked on a Ph.D. in equestrian psychology, studying human-animal relationships in elite equestrian sports. I was enlivened by the work but struggled with isolation and self-doubt. None of my colleagues were human-animal scholars and I was uncomfortable when people asked what my Ph.D. addressed. Although I had put together a convincing rationale for the work, convincing enough to gain institutional approval to conduct the research, deep down I was not convinced of its importance, reflective perhaps of some internalised speciesism. It was during the data collection phase of my Ph.D., interviewing elite equestrians embroiled in the complexities of their hobby-turned-career, that I began to think seriously about the implications of my work.

I am now an academic at a regional university in Australia, my time divided between research, teaching, and administrative work. To thrive in such a role, several characteristics are important. Curiosity, tolerance for uncertainty, attention to detail, and the capacity to think deeply and flexibly are fundamental, particularly where species boundaries are given careful attention. Asking questions is central to all corners of my academic life. Such creativity must be disciplined, however; in writing, thinking, teaching, and designing and conducting research—details matter. Attending to what is absent within academic discourse is as critical as attending to what is present. Flexible working schedules provide a certain level of autonomy and freedom but can also be isolating. I have significant control over my schedule and outputs, but the workload is heavy and in perpetual flux across the academic year. Trying to manage an unevenly dispersed workload can feel like riding a bike down a potholed road, with unexpected hills and descents enlivening the intellectual journey, if you don't fall off your bike entirely.

My most rewarding work tasks contain a common thread: the space to think. This, simultaneously, is the greatest challenge of my work. While thinking can be demanding, the central challenge is not the thinking itself, but being obstreperous enough to make space for intellectual engagement, an aspect of academia that might otherwise very easily feel like a luxury rather than the core business of the academy. As a human-animal researcher and psychology academic, my job is not just to teach psychology, but to extend the discipline and myself into new intellectual, physical, and relational spaces. Creation is as central as critique. Haraway's (2014, para 3) "becoming-with" provides a template for engagement with animals, in and outside the academic praxis. "Becoming-with", she argues, entails an understanding of the fact that "to be a one at all, you must be a many and it's not a metaphor". Solidarity and scholarship, side-by-side. As art expands science, so the human–animal juncture has expanded my experience of what it means to be a psychology academic.

Reference

Haraway, D. (2014). Anthropocene, capitalocene, chthulucene: Staying with the trouble. In *Anthropocene: Arts of living on a damaged planet*. Retrieved May 9, 2014, from http://opentranscripts.org/transcript/anthropocene-capitalocene-chthulucene/

10 From Psychometrics to Animal Metrics

Jean Kirnan

Jean Kirnan, PhD, is a professor of psychology at the College of New Jersey where she has taught for over 30 years. She has a Ph.D. in psychometrics and brings a focus of measurement and assessment to her teaching, consulting, and research. Her research interests include teaching and research on ethical decision making, dog-assisted literacy programs, emotional support animals, and evaluation of mental health education programs.

My introduction to the field of Human-Animal Interactions (HAI) was through my volunteer work as a certified therapy dog handler in my community. I was initially looking for volunteer opportunities for my high school-aged son when another mom shared that she had gotten their dog certified as a therapy dog and her son enjoyed going with her on visits. I home schooled our golden retriever, Nellie, on the tasks required for the Therapy Dog International (TDI) test. Once Nellie passed, we began weekly visits as part of a social hour at an assisted living facility. My son, Pat, was able to complete his volunteer hours with ease. However, when he graduated high school and moved on to college, I realized that I benefited from this work and wanted to continue.

Since 2006, I have certified three additional dogs. Bob and Bailey (Nellie's pups) worked in a dog-assisted literacy program at a local elementary school. Our primary placement was kindergarten, although some years we worked in a special needs classroom. My current therapy dog, Cali, continues to work at the elementary school, but is expanding our horizons by working with a non-profit that focuses on youth mental health education.

My professional training at first seems completely disconnected from HAI. I received my Ph.D. in psychometrics, a field of study dedicated to measurement. I began my career in the business sector designing cognitive ability tests, structured interviews, and biographical inventories for employee selection. After five years, I transitioned into higher education and for the past 34 years have been teaching undergraduate courses in industrial/organizational (I/O) psychology, psychological testing, research, consumer psychology, and psychology of ethics at a college in New Jersey where I am a tenured professor.

After the first year volunteering in the dog-assisted literacy program, I asked the school principal if he was interested in evaluating the program's effectiveness. From this conversation sprang a fruitful collaboration. Along with undergraduates working in my research lab, I studied the literature on Animal Assisted Interventions and HAI in general with a focus on dog-assisted literacy. My students and I analyzed standardized reading scores, conducted interviews, and coded behavioral logs. The result was a tremendous opportunity for me and my students to develop professionally, disseminate our findings in scholarly outlets, and provide evidence to aid the school in the continuance of this program.

Since that time, my students and I have explored other areas of HAI. Current projects include emotional support animals (ESAs) on the college campus as well as working with a new community partner on the effectiveness of a mental health education program that includes therapy dogs. I've also developed a senior seminar on AAI and every semester I present an AAI workshop with a colleague who volunteers in a local equine therapy program.

I hadn't anticipated the unique challenges of conducting research and measuring effectiveness in HAI. My formal training in testing and early professional experiences with employee selection provided a strong foundation in measurement principles, but ingrained in me a rigid and linear way of assessing success. The HAI field includes mixed method research designs and an array of outcome measures including physiological (e.g., heart rate, blood pressure, and hormone levels), standardized test scores (e.g., reading), self-report measures (e.g., anxiety, depression, loneliness), and behavioral change. While I am very comfortable with numbers and test scores, I've had to learn to work with qualitative data (e.g., interviews, focus groups) and anecdotal data such as testimonials. I've learned the limitations of the ".05 probability level" that we strive to achieve in inferential statistics. How do I measure the smile on a child's face as they read to a dog? Or their enthusiasm and determination to master a new book to share with their furry friend? How can I capture the fact that when we enter the "day room" of the assisted living facility, several residents are present, all sitting separately waiting for their turn to pet Nellie—but when we leave an hour later, those same residents are now actively engaged, talking with each other? I find myself simultaneously attempting to apply scientific rigor, but thinking out of the box as I try to develop accurate "animal metrics."

As a college professor and community volunteer I find this field so exciting due to its interdisciplinary nature. I interact with animal trainers, counselors, educators, and health professionals who work with all age and ability groups with a wide array of client needs. So many people can make professional or personal contributions to HAI. For those interested in learning more about this growing field, my strongest recommendation is to observe and participate as often and in as many different venues as possible. Talk to professionals and animal handlers to gain insights and make connections.

Possible areas to investigate:

- Reading dog programs in public libraries or schools
- Animal shelters with volunteer opportunities
- Equine centers that sponsor groundwork (non-riding) and riding therapies
- Colleges that employ therapy dogs for stressful times such as move-in and exams
- Hospitals that employ therapy dogs in both medical and behavioral health facilities

Presenting my first poster on dog-assisted literacy at a professional conference, I explained my background in measurement and evaluation as well as my personal experience as a therapy dog handler to another attendee. She said, "You are so lucky that your research is on something you love." I am so lucky indeed!

11 Rescuing Street Dogs as a Passion and a Way of Being . . .

Úrsula Aragunde Kohl

Úrsula Aragunde Kohl, PsyD, is a clinical psychologist who is committed to working with high-risk communities, creating spaces for social justice and more compassionate ways of living. In 2010, she founded the nonprofit Puerto Rico Alliance for Companion Animals, Inc. (also known as "PR Animals"). Its mission is to educate Puerto Rican communities about compassion, kindness, and responsible guardianship toward all animals. She is also a faculty member at the Universidad Ana G. Mendez, Gurabo Campus, where she developed the first graduate HAI related class.

Ever since I can remember, animals have been part of my life. My mother had a compassionate heart toward street dogs, the Puerto Rican mutts that nobody wanted, so we always rescued them, one dog at a time. For many years, these feelings of compassion, love, and deep respect toward animals have been a curse and a blessing: a curse because it gives me pain to live in a country where animals are poorly treated; a blessing because it drives everything I do today. It has opened many doors and connected me with like-minded people: animal lovers who envision a better and kinder world.

During my graduate courses, I discovered animal-assisted interventions, which led to the development of my doctoral thesis, "Program Design of Animal-Assisted Therapy for Elderly People in Nursing Homes." I graduated with a doctoral degree in clinical psychology and subsequently worked with adolescents utilizing animal-assisted therapy. I proceeded to create a nonprofit organization, the Puerto Rico Alliance for Companion Animals (PR Animals). PR Animals' main mission is to educate Puerto Ricans about having compassion toward and engaging in the responsible guardianship of companion animals. In 2009, I became a faculty member of the graduate psychology program at the Universidad Ana G. Mendez, Gurabo Campus. I developed the first graduate course in Puerto Rico on animal-assisted interventions in health settings. As my main research interest is to investigate how the human-animal bond can optimize human and animal health and wellbeing, I conducted a survey in Puerto Rico to gain a better understanding of the general beliefs about and attitudes toward companion animals.

Results of this work identified people's relationships with companion animals as a source of wellbeing and therapeutic tool in many people's lives.

As a faculty member, my typical day involves teaching, learning, and writing. I teach around four classes per semester and my work schedule is very flexible. During an average week, I am usually at the university for three days from 8am to 3pm, I work from home for one day, and I do volunteer work for the rest of the week (e.g., rescuing, educating, and rehabilitating street dogs). I love to work directly with my companion animals and students. It permits me to collaborate with a diverse group of individuals to create programs that promote compassion and responsibility within Puerto Rico.

As of today, I am also the coordinator for a committee called "Integral Wellbeing through the Human-Animal Relationship" in the Puerto Rico Psychology Association. As the Principal Investigator and Dissertation Director on human-animal interaction research projects, I have helped lay the groundwork for human-animal studies in Puerto Rico. My research has focused primarily on the human-animal bond. Every day in Puerto Rico, we can see and recognize the importance of the development of these relationships in positive and negative terms. The positive aspect is evident in how much we love our pets in our daily lives and interactions, while the negative aspect is evident in the number of stray animals (primarily dogs, cats, and horses) and the unimaginable abuse and negligence of animal companions in many parts of Puerto Rico. To study the relationship between people and their animals is critical for pursuing the path to *everyone's* wellbeing and survival.

My biggest challenge has been figuring out how to enable people (mostly in academia) to understand, first, that the human-animal bond reaches far beyond personal choice and has a direct impact on our wellbeing and, second, that my work is important in spite of the anthropocentric view of most disciplines. The human-animal bond as a research focus and its importance in a social context (e.g., violence, criminality, and addictions) are sometimes trivialized, making it very challenging to use the research to help others understand the bond and the needs of each species so that we can become better guardians of our planet. Yet, as difficult as it sometimes is, promoting kindness and the inclusion of all animals has become part of my lifestyle. The long hours that I spend working are worth it when I consider that I am making a better world for all beings. Knowing that my two main values in life—kindness and courage—are reflected in all aspects of my work makes it very meaningful and less stressful in difficult times.

Being part of the effort to appreciate and cultivate the love that we have for companion animals has allowed me to affect thousands of people and rescue hundreds of animals. It has been an amazing journey. One of the most rewarding aspects of this journey is when people share how grateful they are to know that others also love these special beings as much as they do.

Without a doubt, being a psychologist will give you the opportunity to embark on an amazing journey to help vulnerable groups. However, getting involved in an experience that includes animals in need can broaden your vision and impact. If you love animals, working in the animal welfare community will give you insights into a new dimension of wellbeing, inclusion, and diversity. We are not only helping animals (we will always touch humans with our work too) but also cultivating a society that recognizes the needs of all species without creating a hierarchy of these needs.

It is a job that requires a lot of heart and compassion. Some of the work that must be done comes with the potential for pain and trauma. However, anything that gives you purpose and contributes to the greater good is as valuable as any other endeavor. For me, it has been helping the mutts on my streets in Puerto Rico. For you, it may be a different path, but if it includes animals, I hope we will meet one day.

12 Working in the World of Human–Animal Interaction Research

Beth Lanning

Beth Lanning, PhD, is I am now a professor, the Associate Chair of the Department of Public Health, the Director of the at Baylor University, and a Master Certified Health Education Specialist (MCHES). Her research interest includes human-animal interventions, especially equine-assisted activities and therapy for trauma recovery, veterans with PTSD and depression, children with autism or cerebral palsy, and at-risk youth children.

My love and respect for animals started long before my professional work in public health. My mom bred, trained, and showed golden retrievers and ran obedience schools for years which meant that I grew up around animals. My mom also trained horses and taught me to ride at age 5. I loved riding from an early age and continued riding throughout my childhood. Horses, dogs, and cats were just part of the family. Middle school and high school years can be a difficult time for a lot of people. For me, it was the high school years that proved most difficult. Several situations beyond my control led to me selling my horse before finishing high school. Self-doubt, insecurity, and uncertainty were now part of my life. Then came a special stray dog named Jessie. God brought her into my life at just the right time. I have always believed that God's love shines through His animals, and that was especially true for Jessie. She was my "shadow"; my companion who was always there and happy to spend time with me. I am fortunate to have been able to experience the human-animal bond from an early age and witness how animals have the unique ability to improve a person's quality of life in so many ways.

My professional training is in community/public health. I earned a master of science in education (MSEd) in community health from Baylor University and a PhD in health education from Texas A&M University, and I am an MCHES. In 2000, I accepted a position at Baylor University in the community health program (now the Public Health Program). My pretenure research focused on sexual health and quality of life with a special focus on psychosocial and behavioral health. After being awarded tenure in 2006, I decided to explore bringing my two worlds together: my childhood years with animals and my professional training in public health. I especially wanted to focus on how horses could influence a person's quality of life, yet I found little research in that area. Thus, the birth of my research focus on human-animal interaction (HAI) and the benefits of equine-assisted activities and therapies (EAAT) for various populations.

In public health, HAI fits nicely under the One Health concept. One Health is the unique, dynamic health relationship of human, animal, and environment. It is a concept supported and promoted by the Centers for Disease Control and Prevention (CDC) and the World Health Organization. My work has focused primarily on the psychosocial health benefits of EAAT for military service members and children with autism as well as for other special populations. Because of my role in academia as both a professor and administrator, I also conduct research related to animals and college students. I use the classroom as an opportunity to teach students (many of whom are preparing to work in the healthcare field) about the health benefits of HAI and to encourage them to consider health promotion interventions that include animals in their future work in healthcare and/ or public health.

Currently, there are few public health professionals who conduct research on the psychosocial and physical benefits of HAI within the One Health paradigm. Most public health efforts focus on emerging zoonotic diseases. While this is a critical area in public health, I have enjoyed exploring the social, mental, and physical health benefits of HAI and encourage other public health professionals to do the same. I am fortunate to work in an academic environment that allows me to pursue my work in this area even though it is not a heavily funded area of research. One of my greatest moments of satisfaction occurred sitting in a horse arena with the spouse of a veteran participating in my EAAT study. We cried together as she told me the story of her husband's recovery and how thankful she was for a horse program that she felt "saved" her husband. That is why I conduct research in the area of HAI. It is not about the data or research funding, even though that is important, it is about having an impact on the lives of others and helping improve quality of life—the essence of public health work.

I would encourage public health and other professionals who have an interest in HAI work to learn more about the topic by examining the research literature, attending HAI related conferences such as International Society of Anthrozoology and the Professional Association of Therapeutic Horsemanship International, and visiting organizations that are involved in HAI type work. I would also encourage individuals interested in pursuing HAI related research to take courses in research methods and/or collaborate with others trained in research methods. While many of us have personal stories about the benefits of animals in our lives, it is well designed studies and empirical data that are needed to move human-animal interventions from a novel idea to a best-practice choice.

13 Lessons From a Pioneer in Equine-Assisted Therapies

Arieahn Matamonasa Bennett

Arieahn Matamonasa Bennett, PhD, is an associate professor at DePaul University in Chicago and a licensed psychologist in private practice. Her specialties in clinical practice include connecting to nature and animals (equine-assisted psychotherapy) for healing, growth and change. Her areas of scholarship and expertise include the relationship between societal attitudes towards women, animals and nature; cross-cultural and ethnic minority psychology, the research assessment and practice of psychology with Native American populations, and the exploration of indigenous philosophies, psychologies and cultural healing paradigms

———————

I am a life-long horsewoman whose passion and deep love for horses began in early childhood. I have ridden most of my life in a variety of disciplines and have owned and cared for many horses over the last several decades. I have been actively practicing, teaching and researching equine-assisted therapies since the early 2000s. I am an associate professor at DePaul University and am also the Founder of a private therapy practice that offers equine-assisted therapies. My hope is that by sharing my journey, I can provide valuable guideposts or insights for those interested in entering this complicated but highly rewarding arena. I want to emphasize that equine-assisted therapies are *not* a separate profession, but one in which a *licensed* practitioner partners with an animal in a therapy context within their own therapeutic orientation.

Lesson 1: The Value of Lived-Experience

My lived-experiences with horses helped me to formulate a *working theory* about the value of horse human relationships. These 'lessons' included: 1) learning clear and effective communication, 2) congruency in intent and action, 3) respect and boundaries, 4) taking responsibility for owning and regulating emotions and 5) bonding with horses creates corrective attachment experiences. My 'working theory' resided in my mind during my formal graduate studies, and I thought I might be on the path to *inventing* my own therapeutic intervention. The popular phrase 'hindsight is 20/20' is applicable in that it is now after decades of clinical experience and awareness of the state-of-the–literature that I can see how the important themes from my own experiences reflect major directions within human animal interaction research decades later.

In the early 2000s I was completing my doctoral studies and working with a woman in her mid-life through issues of debilitating depression and anxiety, which today we would quickly identify as trauma from sexual abuse at a young age. In our clinical work, our mutual love of and connection with horses entered the therapy conversation. This client believed that her relationship with a horse throughout her childhood and adolescence was what helped her survive not only the sexual abuse, but also her father's subsequent suicide after the abuse was discovered when she was an adolescent. After our therapy conversations, she brought me the now seminal book *Horses and the Human Heart* by McCormick and McCormick 1997. This book was a gift in so many ways. It affirmed my 'working theories' and inspired me to consider equine-assisted intervention as a legitimate therapeutic tool to add to my 'toolbox.' Based on my knowledge of education and psychology, I began to craft therapeutic and educational experiences that focused on partnering with horses in educational and therapeutic settings. Since that early time, I have completed advanced certifications with EAGALA and have moved on to learn, train, conduct research and partner with practitioners around the world.

Lesson 2: The Need for Training, Mentoring, Supervision and a Learning Community

A well-established principal in psychology is that competency (and excellence) in standards of practice include formal education (certification), *supervised practice* and continuing education. This includes learning *any* therapy modality, including animal assisted interventions. Within therapy modalities there are *many* thought-leaders, theoretical models, organizations and certifications that exist for practitioners, and the same is true for equine-assisted interventions. Additionally, there are strengths, weaknesses and varying levels of *empirically* demonstrated efficacy in all of the current models and none can claim to be the *best* model.

Equine-assisted therapy in all forms is a growing and multidisciplinary modality. There are multiple models/definitions and organizations for professional training/certification. For students researching the field, the lack of a cohesive nomenclature can be frustrating. Students can expect to search terms as varied as therapeutic horsemanship (TH), hippotherapy, equine-assisted psychotherapy (EAP) and equine-assisted learning (EAL). In a study of over 100 EAP practitioners (Matamonasa & Haefner, 2012; Matamonasa, 2015) the lack of a unified field was a theme and was referenced as "the wild west" although organizations such as the Certification Board for Equine

Interaction Professionals (CBEIP) are attempting to establish field-wide certification criteria and ethics.

Lesson 3: Continual Growth Learning and Evolution

Practitioners in equine-assisted therapies are naturally those who feel a strong connection and relationship with horses. The formal field is vast and growing and thus faces numerous challenges. The continually changing landscape and organizations all struggling for their place as *the* model and standard for practice can be frustrating to navigate. Success in this arena requires a strong professional grounding and identity in therapy first, and a willingness to explore multiple models and remain open to new approaches and perspectives. To those interested in the field, I would offer the following:

1. Learn and *master* a theoretical orientation as a platform for your practice whether you practice in the office or want to practice in a stable
2. Utilize theoretical orientation principles as the foundation of equine-assisted interventions
3. Chose an organization to receive training and certification
4. Find mentors to provide guidance and supervision in your therapy practice as you would with any modality
5. Seek continued growth and learning through additional trainings, reading the latest research and taking opportunities to work with others in the field

During the last decade, I have served as a scientific reviewer for Horses and Humans Research Foundation (HHRF) and it has been enlightening and rewarding to review the vast approaches to this field and get a glimpse into all of the interesting ways horses are helping people. It is the power and strength of these lived-experiences that has driven this field forward and will continue to help it evolve in the future.

References

Matamonasa-Bennett, A. (2015). Putting the horse before Descartes: Native American paradigms and ethics in equine assisted therapies. *Business and Professional Ethics Journal*, *33*(4), 23–24.

Matamonasa-Bennett, A., & Haefner, P. (2012). *"How do horses help humans?" Perceptions of therapeutic change among equine-assisted psychotherapy practitioners.* Paper presented at EAGALA National Conference, Santaquin, UT, March.

McCormick, A., & McCormick, M. D. (1997). *Horse sense and the human heart: What horses can teach us about bonding, creativity and spirituality.* Deer-field Beach, FL: Health Communications, Inc.

14 Studying Marine Mammal Behavior—Who Says Academic Careers Are Dry?

Maria Maust-Mohl

Maria Maust-Mohl, PhD, is an associate professor of psychology at Manhattan College, in Riverdale, NY. She received a master's degree from Columbia University in conservation biology and PhD from the Graduate Center of the City University of New York in biopsychology and behavioral neuroscience. Maria has vast experience in the study of animal behavior—in particular, hippos, manatees, dolphins and human perceptions of animals.

For as long as I can remember, I have had a sense of wonder and interest in the behavior of animals, especially marine life. I officially began studying animal behavior as a college student at the University of Arizona where I majored in ecology and evolutionary biology and took classes like animal behavior and marine biology to explore my passion. After my second year, I participated in an Earthwatch program in Hawaii that offered a combination of training and research on dolphin cognition. This two-week program introduced me to greater possibilities involving animal behavior and cognition research. While I was there, I heard about Dr. Irene Pepperberg's parrot cognition lab at the University of Arizona. I did not even realize this lab was at my school because it was in a different department! From the next semester through graduation, I assisted with the care of an African grey parrot and budgerigar in Dr. Pepperberg's lab and worked on several projects studying their cognitive abilities. I also continued searching for different opportunities and received a summer internship at Mote Marine Laboratory involving husbandry and research with two manatees. These experiences allowed me to practice animal behavior work in different settings and develop my research skillset, and helped me decide to pursue graduate school to further explore careers involving animal behavior.

Due to the interdisciplinary nature of animal behavior research, degree programs may be listed under Biology or Psychology departments at different schools. I applied to a range of programs and was accepted into the master's program in conservation biology at Columbia University. I continued to pursue animal behavior research; however I was not yet sure which direction to choose (e.g., field studies, lab studies, zoo research, etc.). I applied for a summer internship at the Bronx Zoo, where I worked in the Ornithology (bird) Department. As an intern, I worked alongside the zookeepers to prepare food, maintain exhibits, and observe the animals. I also conducted an observational study of Lesser Adjutant stork chick behavior, which became the topic of my master's thesis. After graduating, I assisted with several other projects at the Bronx Zoo and I was a zookeeper for a year. Although I loved working at the zoo, I still gravitated toward marine life. I began volunteering in Dr. Diana Reiss's lab at the New York Aquarium where I was introduced to studies of animal communication. While the master's degree provided a greater capacity for research, I did not yet have enough experience to develop independent projects or apply for grants, and so I applied to PhD programs.

Since I already had a background in ecology, I wanted to learn more about the brain and behavior; thus I applied and was accepted to the Biopsychology and Behavioral Neuroscience program at The Graduate Center of the City University of New York (CUNY). My dissertation focused on hippopotamus behavior and communication, but I also contributed to other projects, including a study geared towards developing a museum exhibit on animal minds. For this study, we surveyed people to evaluate their attitudes and knowledge about animal thinking and then used this information to develop an exhibit showcasing scientific discoveries of the animals' cognitive abilities. This project inspired me to become involved in research examining human–animal interactions where I could apply my passion and knowledge of animal behavior in a different way. The PhD program kept me on my toes as I balanced coursework (first two years), research, and teaching (as part of the funding I received). Although I pursued a PhD for research related jobs, I was surprised to discover how much I loved teaching. In fact, I believe this teaching experience was critical to helping me obtain my current job.

Today, I am a full-time, tenured faculty member in the Psychology Department at Manhattan College. Most of my time is spent prepping courses, teaching, grading, and serving on committees. However, there is time outside of class to work on research projects, and winter and summer breaks can be used for data collection, writing manuscripts, and attending conferences. I also enjoy working with students to help them gain research experience and supporting them on independent projects. Collaboration is key to conducting research because of time constraints and limited funding for research travel, equipment, etc. I have been fortunate to partner on various projects with staff at local zoos and faculty in other departments or institutions. I also have had the opportunity to develop a study abroad program where my collaborators and I collect data and students earn college credit, all while snorkeling and observing wild dolphins in the Bahamas.

For people considering careers in animal behavior, my advice is to seek out a variety of volunteer and internship experiences to find the best fit. There are many outlets, such as zoos/aquariums, veterinary clinics, animal shelters, or research centers that involve work with animals. As you search for opportunities, keep an open mind regarding the type of animal, work, and location. These experiences can help you find what interests you the most (e.g., animal care and/or research), form a network of professionals for guidance, and determine if graduate school is the right track. There are also several websites that provide information regarding careers involving animals including:

- www.animaledu.com/student/Careers www.animalbehaviorsociety.org/web/education-careers.php
- www.marinemammalscience.org/for-students/how-to-become-a-marine-mammal-scientist/
- www.aza.org/jobs

15 Academic Pathways Towards HAI

Patricia Pendry

Patricia Pendry, PhD, is an associate professor of human development and graduate faculty member in the Program of Prevention Science at Washington State University. Born and raised in the Netherlands, Patricia teaches graduate and undergraduate courses in research methods, child development, stress and coping, and human development and social policy. She spends most of her time conducting HAI research with graduate and undergraduate students.

I am an associate professor in human development and graduate faculty in the doctoral program in prevention science at Washington State University in Pullman, Wash. While one may not expect an HAI researcher to reside in this discipline, the interdisciplinary nature of prevention science makes it a perfect context in which to study the effects of animal assisted interventions (AAIs) on human and animal participants.

An important theme in my work is that I approach the study of HAI through a 'biobehavioral' lens, which means I examine how biological processes and behavior of humans and animals *interact* in shaping their functioning and wellbeing during AAIs. I am especially interested in understanding the effects of university-based AAIs in preventing the negative consequences of social and academic stress in youth and college students and the role biological processes may play in shaping these effects.

Focusing on equine- and canine-assisted interventions, I conduct randomized controlled trials in real-life settings to examine their effects on activity of the part of the brain active in regulating responses to stress, the Hypothalamic Pituitary Adrenal (HPA) axis. I do this by collecting samples of saliva, which are analyzed for changes in cortisol production to examine whether interaction with animals affects HPA-axis activity and ultimately, functioning in various developmental domains (e.g., socioemotional, cognitive, physical).

Rather than focusing only on the human side of the HAI equation, I also analyze characteristics and behavior of the animals we work with by video recording AAI sessions and activities. My students and I carefully code the behaviors of all parties involved—animals, handlers and clients—to better understand what constitutes *high-quality* interaction, and how to promote interactions that are beneficial for humans and animals alike.

As such, my research spans across basic and applied approaches, and draws from literatures of human development; developmental psychoneuroendocrinology; psychometrics; anthrozoology; animal assisted intervention; animal science and behavior; and program design, implementation and evaluation.

Day-to-Day Rewards

As a faculty member, I divide my time between conducting research on HAI; teaching a variety of graduate and undergraduate courses; mentoring students; and providing service to professional associations, my university, college, and department, and residents of Washington state. Some of the most rewarding parts of my job are that I have the opportunity to interact with animals on a regular basis. This is extremely enjoyable—not just because I like animals, but also because it is so much fun to see the effects of HAI on all parties involved, including AAI facilitators. I feel very fortunate that I get to engage with wonderful people who dedicate themselves to facilitating meaningful and impactful interactions between humans and animals. It is an environment that creates positive feelings, generativity towards others and awareness about our day-to-day presence and opportunity for connection. It is also a nice antidote to the stress, negativity and material tendencies to which so many of us fall victim.

In addition, I thoroughly enjoy working with students in and outside the classroom. In fact, I like nothing more than successfully bringing my students into the field by getting them excited about research and practice of HAI related endeavors. In particular, I love being a mentor to my graduate students with whom I work closely on a daily basis as they move through the phases of graduate study to becoming junior colleagues.

Challenges

As with any career, being an academic comes with specific challenges, including the pressure to obtain external funding, publish frequently, be a great teacher and mentor, and provide impactful service. The pressure and the desire to succeed result in a substantially greater than 40-hour workweek on a regular basis. That said, as long as you keep juggling—and catching—lots of different balls in the air, this career is extremely rewarding.

Pathway Towards HAI

People are often surprised to find out that the path that led me to my career in HAI and academe was extremely circuitous. I first attended college in

Netherlands where I was raised, 'dabbling' in law and public affairs without much conviction or enthusiasm. After moving to the US, I started taking psychology classes, which ignited my passion for understanding links between stress, physiology, behavior and health. This led me to obtain a psychology degree as an adult student, followed by a PhD in human development and social policy, both from Northwestern University, followed by a tenure track appointment at WSU.

Although much of my graduate study was focused on examining contributions of stress to dysregulation of HPA axis activity, I became curious about the possible ways to 'undo' the negative effects of stress exposure on physiological dysregulation. It wasn't until I engaged in a pen-and-pencil brainstorming exercise about possible stress management interventions that I remembered the childhood joys of spending weekends at a local barn where interactions with horses, dogs, cats, goats, chickens and potbelly pigs became the highlight of my week. It was those memories, combined with a passion for research that led me to study the efficacy of AAIs. I am very grateful for receiving generous grants from the National Institutes of Health, Washington State University and MARS/Waltham that have allowed me to conduct randomized controlled trials on the effects of HAI on humans and animals and establish a record of scholarship.

16 Civic Engagement of Students Through Human-Animal Interactions

Alina Simona Rusu

Alina Simona Rusu is a biologist and psychologist who received her PhD in natural sciences from the University of Zürich, Switzerland. Currently, Alina is an associate professor at the Department of Special Education (School of Psychology and Sciences of Education, Babeş-Bolyai University, Cluj-Napoca, Romania), where she teaches several classes. Alina is also the main coordinator of the postgraduate program "Animal Assisted Therapy and Activities for Persons with Special Needs", which is currently the only existing academic program in the field in Romania.

I am an associate professor in the Special Education Department, School of Psychology and Sciences of Education at Babeş-Bolyai University (BBU), located in the North-Western part of Romania. I have a double degree in psychology and biology and a PhD in natural sciences (animal behavior) from the University of Zurich, Switzerland. While doing my PhD research on the social behavior of wild house mice from 2000 to 2004, I had the chance to come across the field of Animal-Assisted Therapy by interacting with one of the professors in the Department of Animal Behavior, Dennis C. Turner. At that time, Dr. Turner was the President of the International Association of Human-Animal Interaction Organizations (IAHAIO) and Founder of the Institute for Applied Ethology and Animal Psychology, Switzerland.

It was a Friday evening in 2003, when, while in the lab collecting behavioral data on mice for one of my studies, I heard the sound of many dog paws and cheerful human voices heading toward the seminar room of our Animal Behavior Department. I soon discovered that those eight people and their fluffy dogs were attending a workshop on applied values of human-animal interactions. At that time I had no idea that animals can be included in clinical or educational practice, so I returned to my mice, but I did not stay with them too many years after that Friday. Something had definitely changed in me that day in terms of professional interests and trajectory.

Ten years later, back in Romania, after I completed an online training on Animal Assisted Therapy and Activities offered by Pet Partners in collaboration with University of North Texas, US, I became the main coordinator of a postgraduate program "Animal Assisted Therapy and Activities for Persons with Special Needs", hosted by BBU. This program is currently the only form of animal-assisted intervention academic training in Romania. Since 2013, the program has attracted more than 500 graduates from various professional fields such as: veterinary medicine, psychology, special education, physical rehabilitation, social work, primary and gymnasium education, and human medicine. In addition to this program, I also teach an animal psychology course for undergraduate students in psychology. Following the example of good practices offered years ago by Dr. Turner, in my animal psychology class, I encourage students to include their companion animals in the class activities and we always reflect in a meaningful manner on the benefits and risks associated to animal presence in the educational context. Veterinarian specialists are often invited to our classes, as well as accredited animal-assisted therapy teams, dog trainers and feline behavior counselors, so the students have the possibility to discover various animal-oriented professional directions. Even if they do not become themselves experts in animal-assisted interventions, students become aware that they can collaborate with the existent practitioners, researchers and educators in the area of human-animal interactions.

Ongoing Projects and Recommendations

While an impressive body of research exists supporting the psycho-physiological benefits of human-animal interactions (HAI) on several aspects of human quality of life, I was happy to discover that there are studies indicating that the civic skills and prosocial attitudes, which are important components of social health, can be enhanced by positive HAI, especially by Humane Education programs (Komorosky & O'Neal, 2015; Arkow, 2015; Rusu, 2017). Programs that are addressing community needs in terms of HAI, such as prevention of abuse toward animals and promoting responsible ownership, have been reported to positively impact the level of empathy toward animals and toward humans of students involved in these programs (Tedeschi, Fitchett, & Molidor, 2005; Rusu & Davis, 2018). Empathy is considered a crucial component of civic engagement (Komorosky & O'Neal, 2015). I do consider that being aware of this type of research is important in building the social awareness of students and facilitating valuable networking with colleagues around the world working with volunteers and animals. Therefore, in my interactions with my students, whenever we are involved in community-oriented activities promoting the responsible ownership or targeting the awareness towards the benefits of animal presence in various institutions (special education schools, hospitals, penitentiaries etc.), I do encourage the usage of reflective practices that are based on compassion and empathy building, i.e. empathy towards people, animals and environment. In line with this, like other colleagues in the field, I support the idea that the inclusion of animals (from animal presence to animal-assisted therapy and social veterinary medicine) in service-learning activities has the potential to provide an enhanced educational environment for civic involvement, personal growth and development of social competencies not only in students in animal-related professions, but also in other professions focusing on *helping others*.

References

Arkow, P. (2015). Animal therapy on the community level: The impact of pets on social capital. In *Handbook of animal-assisted therapy. Foundations and guidelines for animal-assisted interventions* (4th ed.). Cambridge, MA: Elsevier.

Komorosky, D., & O'Neal, K. K. (2015). The development of empathy and prosocial behavior through humane education, restorative justice, and animal-assisted programs. *Contemporary Justice Review, 18*, 395–406.

Rusu, A. S. (2017). Constructing healthy experiences through human-animal interactions for autistic children and their families: Implications for research and education. In J. Yip (Ed.), *Autism—paradigms and clinical applications* (pp. 269–290). London: Tech Publisher, ISBN 978-953-51-5013-8.

Rusu, A. S., & Davis, R. (2018). *Civic engagement of students through human-animal interactions: Ideas for an interdisciplinary service learning-based curriculum*. CIEA 2018 Proceedings of the Fifth International Conference on Adult Education, Iasi, Romania, pp. 583–590.

Tedeschi, P., Fitchett, J., & Molidor, C. E. (2005). The incorporation of animal-assisted interventions in social work education. *Journal of Family Social Work, 9*, 59–77.

17 An HAI Love Story

A Couple Collaborates as Teachers and Researchers Exploring Our Connection to Animals

Dieter and Netzin Steklis

Dieter Steklis, PhD, is a professor in the School of Animal and Comparative Biomedical Sciences at the University of Arizona, with an affiliated faculty appointment in psychology, Program in Ethology and Evolutionary Psychology. Dieter has also held several leadership positions in the private not-for-profit sector and conducts research (in collaboration with his wife Netzin Steklis) on mountain gorilla behavior and conservation.

Netzin Steklis, PhD, is an associate professor in the School of Animal and Comparative Biomedical Sciences at the University of Arizona. Netzin has studied a variety of nonhuman primates in captive and wild settings, in particular the ecology, social behavior, and conservation of wild mountain gorillas in Rwanda. She has co-developed and teaches courses with her husband (Dr. H. Dieter Steklis), including Human and Animal Interrelationships, animal ethology and ethics, and primate captive management and welfare.

This is a story of a scientist couple brought together by their love of animals. Our complementary backgrounds and professional training make us a strong multidisciplinary couple. Netzin has degrees and training in anthropology, biology and primatology, ecology and evolutionary biology, and evolutionary psychology. Dieter's degrees and training comprise biological anthropology, primatology, comparative anatomy, behavioral biology, and neurobiology. We pursued primatology independently, with both of us studying primates in the wild, and Dieter adding considerable experimental laboratory work (hormone and neurobiological studies) working with several monkey species. It's no accident that we met at a primatology conference and sealed our destiny together.

Our long-term, shared interests in animals naturally led us to our present involvement in the HAI (human-animal interaction) field. Although each of us concentrated on primate research, we explored the interdisciplinary aspects of primatology—animal behavior, ecology, and evolutionary-comparative studies (traditionally known as ethology) of a variety of mammals. The HAI field by its nature is interdisciplinary, attracting scientists from diverse disciplines (e.g., clinical psychology, animal behavior, zoology, anthropology) to form collaborative research teams. This realization led to our founding in 2014 of the Human–Animal Interaction Research Initiative (HAIRI) at the University of Arizona as a way to attract students and faculty from different university departments to collaborate on HAI research.

Our group's HAI research projects cover a broad range of topics. For brevity, we'll describe the projects in terms of questions each project tries to answer. For example: Does dog ownership among the elderly lower inflammation and improve health? Do therapy dog visits to an Intensive Care Unit reduce stress among nursing staff? How has our long evolutionary history together with both domesticated and wild animals shaped our psychology and theirs? Are human attitudes and feelings toward other animals predictable from human personality or do they comprise a distinct component of human psychology? Each of these projects brings together experts from several disciplines.

We are professors at the University of Arizona, which means that a good portion of each day is spent teaching; the rest is spent working with students and faculty colleagues on our research projects. We are fortunate in that we have been able to design our own courses and co-teach them as a couple. For example, we built an introductory level course called "Human and Animal Interrelationships" that covers the history of the myriad relationships between humans and various nonhuman animal species and how particular kinds of human–animal relationships (e.g., domesticated, prey, predator, pets) have over time changed both humans and animals biologically, psychologically, and culturally. We stress how certain domesticated animals, such as dogs and horses, crucially influenced the course of human evolution and the course of civilization.

Importantly, our teaching and scholarship is driven by our passion for understanding and working with animals, and so we take every opportunity to spend time observing and studying animals. At home, this includes our own animals (which over the years have included dogs, horses, chickens, cockatiels, hamsters, and chameleons), but we also get away frequently to observe and study wild animals, such as monkeys, chimps, and gorillas in Rwanda, Africa, as well as wolves and ravens. These experiences refuel our passion and continue to shape our thinking and the content of our teaching and research.

After reading all this, you may well think, "Wow, this is the dream job!" Not so fast. Like any job or career, there are challenges and downsides. For one, academic positions are few and highly competitive, and they require an advanced degree (at least a master's) and often a record of established and promising scholarship, research, and publication. This means investing heavily in time and money resources up front in the hope of a later payoff. And if you do get an academic position, be prepared for continued long dedicated hours of work. In our experience, workdays are neither 8 hours long, nor do they exclude weekdays or holidays. In other words, our "work" naturally permeates our personal lives. We joke that our "dates" as a married couple are long intellectual discussions over a glass of wine about some animal related news story or new research project. For some, this kind of life with no clear separation between work and home life may be understandably stressful and unacceptable, even if the work fully engages one's passion and interests. This is important to know about yourself before entering the HAI field through an academic career rather than being surprised by it. Fortunately, this is not a conflict for us, probably because our seemingly endless curiosity about the animal world attracted us to the profession and quite naturally shaped how we spend our time professionally and personally (even though we like to complain about being overworked and underpaid). On the plus side, we feel personally fulfilled because we have made it a rule to include our children in all our professional activities, and because through our teaching and research, we can help to improve human relationships to other animals, especially by enhancing the welfare of animals in our care (e.g., factory-farmed animals, zoo animals). HAI is a relatively new and growing field, with many and diverse career opportunities, that can be entered from multiple degree programs and disciplines (e.g., go to this publication to see which HAI career best fits you: Erdman, P., LaFollette, M.R., Steklis, N.G., Steklis, H.D., Germone, M.M., and Kogan, L. Guide to Human-Animal Interaction Education. Human Animal Interaction Bulletin 6:37–46, 2018).

18 An Academic Career Based on What I Love

People, Animals, and Health

Cindy C. Wilson

Cindy C. Wilson, BS, MS, Phd, CHES. (ret), is a professor in the Department of Family Medicine Uniformed Services University of the Health
Sciences (USUHS) in Bethesda, Maryland, USA. Cindy has decades of
research experience focusing on the therapeutic value of companion animals
(CAs) in college students, elderly persons, and normal populations. She has
served on review panels for the NIH as well as foundations in the areas of
health and education.

It all started with the need to euthanize 10,000 animals at a metropolitan county Humane Society. My best friend and working colleague was
interviewing for the Executive Director position and was asked by a board
member if she would have any problem making these decisions. She quickly
excused herself from candidacy and hurried to my home to debrief and
develop a plan for our future. The plan we developed combined the three
things that were (and still are) most important to us. We wanted to work
with each other—knowing our approaches to research would complement
each other (she has a Ph.D. in social work and is very detail oriented, and
I have an M.S. in Animal Science and a Ph.D. in Public Health and like to
develop the conceptual framework of researchable questions). We wanted
to work with biopsychosocial aspects of aging and we wanted to involve
animals. By the time my friend left that day, we had outlined an approach to
develop a state-of-the art review of CAs and the elderly. Little did we know
that our plan would evolve into a professional collaboration that would last
for more than 44 years.

After completing my doctorate in public health, I initially taught public
health courses at a small liberal arts university. Subsequently, I worked as
a health consultant developing health education programs for a national
health systems agency. From there I went on to work for a regional public
health department and directed a child health initiative. Within a short
period of time, I moved to the position of assistant dead for research at a
major institution of higher education where my responsibilities included
resource development, grants acquisition, research policy development,

coordination of corporate contacts, and assisting faculty with grant writing. Following this position, I became the Health Administration Manager for a Robert Wood Johnson foundation grant to the State of Missouri and the University of Missouri-Columbia to regionalize all maternal and child health services within the state. After this experience, I taught two years of both undergraduate and graduate courses at Arizona State University. At that point, I was recruited to the Uniformed Services University of the Health Sciences (USUHS) as the Research Director of Family Medicine and ten years later, implemented the first faculty development program at the University.

Throughout my career, I found that I used my program development and project management skills more than any others. Regardless of whether I was running a program or a grant or developing materials and syllabi for courses, setting goals and measurable objectives were essential. These skills were invaluable, whether I was writing about the value of CAs with the elderly, developing the first pet placement program in subsidized housing, assessing the psycho-bio-social impact of a dog on college students and military caregivers, or most recently, the psycho-bio-social impact of a service dog on a service member.

Since I have spent most of my career as an academic, my time is divided into teaching, research, and service. Since I have been a professor at USUHS, my teaching focuses on faculty, fellows, and residents. My research tends to go in two directions. First, clinical research that helps junior faculty reach their promotion requirements. Second, my own research that looks at various aspects of human animal interactions and how those interactions impact a participant's health (defined broadly).

The most rewarding parts of my position are: (1) when a learner has that "ah ha" moment of understanding; (2) when I am able to take an idea from its inception to operationalizing it into a hypothesis, research aims, and objectives; and ultimately, when I can see the impact of HAIs on study participants. The surprising element related to my research on HAIs is that I can volunteer with any number of content related community organizations (e.g., Humane Society, Pets on Wheels, Warrior Canine Connection, etc.) and have it "count" as a service activity for promotion and tenure.

There are several challenges in my work. These include the enormous about of paperwork because of Department of Defense regulations and requirements regarding research in this setting. In additional, because many of my collaborators are military personnel, they are only at the University for a short period of time. This makes longitudinal research more challenging.

Another challenge relates to personnel changes in the research offices that often result in contradictory guidance regarding our studies. Lastly, the number of institutional review boards (IRBs) to which we are accountable increases based on the number of hospitals and how many services (Army, Navy, Public Health, etc.) are involved. Another challenge is that there is no limit to the number of hours in your work week and you will often work at home as much as in your office. However, there is great autonomy in what you do.

Core competencies needed for an academic position include a solid knowledge in content, research methodology, and statistics. Essential to your success is the ability to read and understand material across disciplines. In additional, you must be able to lead a project if you are to succeed in academe. The last bit of advice that I would offer regarding your career path is to determine what is most important you in terms of work and to build a strong, collegial network of colleagues. The rest will sort itself out.

Part II

Academic—With Clinical Work

19 Insights From a Late Bloomer in the Field of Human–Animal Interactions

John-Tyler Binfet

John-Tyler Binfet, PhD, is an associate professor in the Faculty of Education at the University of British Columbia, Okanagan campus. He is a leading researcher on school kindness, and his work strives to uncover how children, adolescents, and educators understand kindness in school and what they do to demonstrate kindness. In addition to his work on kindness, John-Tyler is the Founder and Director of UBC's dog therapy program "B.A.R.K."

I have, perhaps, an unusual trajectory to landing a job in academia at a research-intensive university where I am a researcher in the fields of human-animal interactions (HAI) and child development. At the ripe age of 48, I began a tenure-track position at the University of British Columbia (UBC), having completed a Ph.D. as a young person but having had my career take a backseat to that of my spouse. As a former public school teacher and counsellor, I was well versed in all things education and having a Ph.D. in educational and counselling psychology and special education helped me in landing a fast-paced job at an age when many folks are beginning to wind down their careers. Trained in adolescent moral development, little did I know the freedom I had to carve out new and innovative research topics as a new faculty member. Now, as a tenured, associate professor I maintain two research streams: 1) exploring the effects of canine-assisted interventions (CAIs) on undergraduate student well-being; and 2) exploring children and adolescents' conceptualizations of kindness at school. I publish almost equally on both topics and run an alternate cycle whereby one year I submit a grant on one topic and conduct a study on the other topic and then switch the following year.

Having been a community handler with my own therapy dog back in California, I was familiar with CAIs and the ins and outs of volunteering with my dog. Upon arrival to UBC, I'd bring my dog with me to the office and as I'd walk across campus to get coffee each morning, I would be besieged by students—students who, for the most part, barely acknowledged me—but immediately began talking to and interacting with my dog. These students would eventually look up and with tear-filled eyes tell me that as much as they missed their parents, they missed their dog more. I knew then that there was a strong need for a canine program on campus to meet students' social and emotional needs.

This was the beginning of UBC's "Building Academic Retention through K9s" or B.A.R.K. program (www.barkubc.ca), a robust on-campus program with over 60 credentialed dog-handler teams. We now have two different weekly in-person programs to support student well-being, a virtual canine comfort program, and a program at the local police detachment to support officer and staff stress reduction. The B.A.R.K. office employs a part-time program coordinator and several research assistants, and offers mentorship to 30 undergraduate student volunteers each year.

In my role as the Director of B.A.R.K., my time is spent overseeing operations and the delivery of programs, supervising personnel, and designing and running studies. As UBC runs on a semester system, B.A.R.K. programming is especially busy in the fall and winter after which we turn our attention to the screening and training of volunteer dog-handler teams. We credential our own teams using a rigorous process developed in B.A.R.K. that involves a handler orientation, practice training sessions, a formal assessment, and an internship before teams can be accepted for work on behalf of B.A.R.K. We do no recruitment of volunteers and typically have a waitlist of potential handlers seeking to participate in our screening process.

The most rewarding aspects of my job are grounded in the interactions I'm privileged to witness and be a part of each day—interactions where a psychologically fragile student who is withdrawn comes to life during interactions with the B.A.R.K. dogs. Post-hoc notes or emails, sometimes long after a student has graduated, telling me of the role the dogs played in their life remind me of the important work I'm doing. Challenges in running a large program include preventing overcrowding in sessions, monitoring student and canine welfare, and running studies whose findings hold potential to advance our scientific understanding of the role dogs play in promoting well-being.

Who Is Well-Suited to Doing This Kind of Work?

One of the challenges for researchers working in the field of HAI, especially for those who investigate the effects of interactions between humans and animals, is that they must have expertise and scientific proficiency in both human and animal domains. The complexities of designing and running interventions studies require straddling two distinct, yet mutually-informing worlds. One must have a keen interest in, and strong foundational knowledge of both humans and animals, and this may not be necessarily easy to cultivate or come by. In addition, researchers must also have in-depth knowledge of research methodology (typically initiated in one's undergraduate and graduate coursework). Last, I feel strongly that researchers working in HAI must have a sense of what it is like to be a volunteer in a program (e.g., a canine handler in a CAI) so they are able to understand the nuanced behaviors and interactions that can inform policy guidelines around program delivery.

Undergraduate students keen on working in the field of HAI are encouraged to gain experience through volunteering—whether on-campus or in community-based programs. Both undergraduate and graduate students are also encouraged to volunteer for research projects conducted on their campus, either as volunteers or as hired research assistants.

20 Labracadabra! The Magic of Animal-Assisted Social Work

Yvonne Eaton-Stull

Yvonne Eaton-Stull, DSW, is an associate professor of social work at Slippery Rock University in Pennsylvania. She is a licensed clinical social worker and specializes in crisis intervention, forensic social work, and animal-assisted social work and provides clinical intervention to children and adults. She has three therapy dogs and actively provides animal-assisted therapy in various mental health facilities. She is also a member of HOPE AACR where she provides animal-assisted crisis response following crises and disasters throughout the United States.

Once upon a time, I had a supervisor who challenged me to "increase client attendance in groups". I thought, well, I would go if there was a dog there, so I asked my supervisor about animal-assisted groups. She then tasked me with putting a proposal together to present to the board of directors. I compiled research, designed a group for adults with depression, presented to the board, and got a green light. This began my journey into animal-assisted social work. For several years, I worked in this outpatient mental health clinic providing social work to both kids and adults. I was able to register my Labrador retriever, Maggie, as a therapy dog and ran groups on anger management, self-esteem, depression, and post-traumatic stress disorder, just to name a few. I wanted to demonstrate the benefits of these groups, so I was sure to collect pre- and post-test measures. These groups were amazingly successful and what was truly rewarding was seeing the changes in clients! One adult in a depression group shrieked in terror as Maggie and I entered the room. Mortified, I thought my co-facilitator had forgotten to explain there was a dog in the group. The client responded that she truly wanted to attend and hoped to overcome her fear of dogs. So with some quick thinking, we re-arranged the circle of chairs placing her chair in the corner away from any contact with the dog. Over the course of the ten weeks, she slowly moved her chair in the circle, progressed from letting the dog pass in front of her to petting her. At the conclusion of the group, she posed for a picture hugging the dog so that she could "hang it on my refrigerator to show my family that I overcame my fear".

Throughout my early career providing animal-assisted social work, I was also doing volunteer work, providing animal-assisted crisis response with my two Labrador retrievers. One such deployment, to Virginia Tech University after the mass shooting, opened up some new doors. Upon returning from this tragedy, I discovered a job opening as the Director of a college counseling center. Since I had enjoyed my interactions with college students, I decided to apply. I credit Maggie with landing this job for me because the college was very interested in her work and hoped to have her as an added benefit. Soon after starting this job, we created "Mondays with Maggie" where from 4–5pm every Monday students could just stop in to visit with the therapy dog. This was a great way to increase student comfort with the counseling center in case they needed services in the future. For eight years, Maggie and my other dog, Zeus, accompanied me about once a week to support the students on campus in individual therapy, homesickness groups, and post-suicide intervention.

While working at the college counseling center, I was also working on completing my doctorate degree and choose to do my dissertation on animal-assisted crisis response. Upon completing my dissertation and earning my doctorate, I wanted to move into academia full time. I was fortunate to land my current dream job, teaching social work at Slippery Rock University! Part of what makes this such a great job is the progressive nature and encouragement of my department. I have been able to develop new courses on animal-assisted intervention (AAI) and crisis intervention where therapy dogs are integrated into classes. I also collaborated with the recreational therapy department to develop a minor in AAI. In more recent years, I assisted in the development of a master's in social work program that includes an animal-assisted certificate. Meanwhile, I am encouraged to pursue my passion—providing AAI in prisons (with my current dog Chevy). My recent research has included the provision of groups (with and without therapy dogs) on stress management, self-harm, grief, and post-partum issues to incarcerated individuals. It is so rewarding to include students in this work and share the value that therapy animals bring to the lives of clients. It is equally exciting to add to the evidence-base of this invaluable intervention.

There is no doubt that this specialty area is growing and in need of trained, experienced practitioners. Those who are considering a career in this field are encouraged to get involved: you might consider training and registering your own dog as a therapy dog; or work alongside canine teams providing comfort and support following disasters and crises by getting involved with such organizations as HOPE Animal-Assisted Crisis Response (www.hope aacr.org). I have also found that many therapy dog teams are willing to (with permission of the agency) allow students to shadow and observe their work, so contacting therapy dog handlers near you is another opportunity to gain knowledge and experience.

This work is not only a career, it is a lifestyle filled with loving dogs. For me, this career path has been a wonderful, surprising journey whereby I have been able to see the magic my dogs offer to my clients. My only regret is that I didn't do this sooner.

21 Human–Animal Bond in Colorado (HABIC) at Colorado State University

Helen Holmquist-Johnson

Helen Holmquist-Johnson, PhD, is the Director of Human-Animal Bond in Colorado (HABIC) at Colorado State University. Her expertise includes designing, implementing, and evaluating animal-assisted interventions (AAI), and support services including training AAI volunteers and clinicians to administer interventions and use data to refine treatments. She has partnered with many federal agencies, private evaluation firms, and county and state departments to design and implement AAI interventions.

———

I am the Director of Human-Animal Bond in Colorado (HABIC)—and HAI Center housed in the School of Social Work at Colorado State University. HABIC has approximately 150 volunteers who provide AAI with their certified HABIC animals in various treatment settings including schools, hospitals, hospices, mental health treatment centers, and long-term care facilities. HABIC is unique because we provide the training, screening, and insurance required to volunteer in a wide variety of settings. Our volunteer Human-Animal teams typically spend one hour per week working with clients and professionals (i.e., social workers, psychologists, occupational therapists, speech therapists) on therapeutic goals. In addition to AAI programs, we are currently creating an online certificate program for people wanting to learn more about the Human-Animal Bond and how to conduct AAI and relevant research.

My path leading to my current position was far from linear. In my early college education, as a lifelong animal lover, I was set on becoming a veterinarian. However, once enrolled in biology and other animal sciences courses, I quickly realized that working with sick animals was, for me, quite emotionally challenging. I knew my path would be different—that I wanted to work with healthy animals. I wanted to combine helping people with healthy animals. It was in that pursuit that I discovered the profession of social work. The core values of social work, specifically the person in the environment and strengths perspective, have always resonated with me.

After graduating with my BS in psychology I decided to explore a master's in social work (MSW) program. I tracked down the Council on Social

Work Education Directory of Accredited programs—a list of all potential programs of study. Flipping through the program catalog I saw, for the very first time, three words linked together. Listed under the heading Colorado State University master's of social work were the words "Human-Animal Bond". My eyes stopped reading and my fate was sealed. That's exactly what I wanted to study, so I decided to pursue my MSW at Colorado State University.

After observing HABIC therapy sessions as a student, and writing grants in the HABIC office, I decided that I wanted to become even more involved. My husband and I were newly married with our own house so the timing was right for us to get a puppy. I had my heart set on a black Labrador retriever. I carefully researched pedigrees and breeders with therapy work, specifically HABIC, in mind. My husband I were both graduate students at the time, but somehow we scraped together enough money to make the deposit for a puppy. Several weeks later the breeder called to tell us she had nine yellow puppies. I was disappointed that my black pup was not in the litter, but we had made our deposit and so reluctantly we went to visit the litter—just to be sure we wanted to wait for a black pup.

Well, we all know how this scenario ends. Once again my fate was sealed as we brought home Aspen—the yellow pup who stole my heart. She grew into a skilled HABIC dog who craved the attention of children. I have so many stories about those years, but one of our most impactful moments came when a young boy who was non-verbal and living with autism spectrum disorder spoke his first words out loud to Aspen. We were awestruck!

Words cannot adequately express how important this work is to me. We, as social workers, know what it means and what it takes to speak on behalf of those who do not have a voice, whether it's a dog, or people struggling to have agency in their own lives. I consider animal-assisted therapy work, and the promotion of the human animal bond, to be my life's work.

Career Options

The career options for social workers who are interested in combining their work with animals have increased dramatically over the last decade. Because AAI is a non-billable service, most of this work is done under the auspices of non-profit organizations; therefore, it is important to gain skills related to non-profit management. These skills include working with volunteers, donors, a board or advisory committee, fiscal management, fundraising, grant writing, and program evaluation. With passion and in-depth knowledge of your organization you will be capable of attracting donors and community supporters who are interested in partnering with you to fulfill the mission of the organization. The American Evaluation Association (www.eval.org) is a valuable professional association for anyone who is looking to gain skills in the area of program evaluation. Look for degree programs that offer a certificate in non-profit management or give credit for electives courses from schools of business or other departments teaching this curriculum.

Some current and exciting career and research opportunities that illustrate the intersection of social work and HAI include: how best to co-shelter people with animals in temporary housing and during natural disasters, grief and loss of pets, training service animals to help people with psychological or physical disabilities, the link between animal abuse and other forms of violence, ensuring welfare for animals providing assisted interventions, and providing support to underserved pet owners or those who are experiencing homelessness. Excellent resources to pursue are: the Human–Animal Bond Research Institute (HABRI) https://habri.org/ and Veterinary Social Work at The University of Tennessee, Knoxville https://vetsocialwork.utk.edu/, and Animals and Society www.animalsandsociety.org/.

22 Mutual Rescue

From Multiple Sclerosis to Working With Therapy Dogs in Education

Diana Peña Gil

Diana Peña Gil graduated with an MS in pedagogy from the Complutense University of Madrid, and is currently working on her PhD as a research staff in training at the Faculty of Education. Diana also collaborates with different companies in the design and evaluation of programs of animal-assisted interventions to improve the quality of life of people.

It is curious how I began to be interested in the effects that animals, specifically dogs, can have on people. I was 19 years old at the time, scheduled to take the competency test needed to obtain my credentials to do canine assisted search and rescue work in the mountains. One afternoon, however, I started feeling dizzy and seeing double. Two weeks later I got the diagnosis: I had multiple sclerosis. This diagnosis nullified the possibility of entering the rescue association, so I found myself without a future and with a disease that I knew little about.

It was during this low time that my parents decided to give me the opportunity I had long desired: let me adopt a dog. I had always wanted a dog, but my parents always refused saying it was a big responsibility to have a well-trained dog. Over the years, I have come to understand and appreciate their decisions.

Visiting animal shelters, looking for my dog, fate intervened and Skot appeared. He was my first therapy dog, a mix breed of German shorthaired pointer and Great Dane who radically changed my life. The first months were what marked my destiny. I realized how Skot impacted me, making me more social, cheerful, and even more physically healthy. As a result, I started reading books and researching.

I decided to return to the academic world and study pedagogy and the benefits of human-animal interactions (HAI). I also took advantage of other forms of training including dog-assisted therapy, dog behavior, and animal welfare—learning and deepening my appreciation for the HAI field. It was during this time that I discovered Skot's potential as a therapy dog. He had always loved being surrounded by people, and his size and temperament were perfect for the job.

Together with Skot, I began volunteering at animal shelters and dog-assisted therapy programs. After that, I had my first HAI-related paying job opportunity. I formed an association of dog-assisted interventions with some colleagues and for a year we facilitated HAI programs in nursing homes, schools, and special education centers. But I needed more; I wanted a deeper understanding of human-animal interactions. I returned to the university, and after completing a master's degree in educational guidance I began working on my doctorate degree in education. I am currently about to finish my PhD, and am proud to be the first person in Spain to include therapy dogs within university classrooms.

My day-to-day schedule involves teaching every morning, accompanied by my new therapy dog (Skot retired in 2019). In my classes, I encourage students to see human-animal interactions as an educational possibility. In the afternoons I work on research and train dogs. It is a fantastic schedule, although sometimes it is exhausting.

I love my current position. I have been able to successfully combine the two things that I like most in the world—education and dogs. However, not everything is positive, and there are significant challenges. Spain is a country that, although advancing in the field of human-animal interactions, still has a long way to go. Bureaucratic struggles, financial problems, and job stability are three prevalent challenges.

When people ask me about career decisions, I always answer them with another question: will the proposed path reward and satisfy you? It is not an easy question and it varies according to each person. If someone wants to find out if the area of human-animal interactions is something they should pursue, my recommendations are the following:

- Research the subject and reach out to the people in the field who interest you. You will be surprised how many people will respond positively.
- Volunteer for an animal shelter and in an animal-assisted intervention program. You will find a different vision.
- Take time to think about what you could do every day of your life without getting tired or bored and if it includes animals.
- Do not give up; realize that the road can be hard, but the rewards can be plentiful.

23 Getting in the HABIT

Bringing Animal Assisted Interventions to Victims of Crime

Bethanie A. Poe

Bethanie A. Poe, PhD, LMSW, graduated from the University of Tennessee's (UT) College of Social Work's PhD program and was a fellow in UT's Veterinary Social Work program where she helped to develop the Veterinary Social Work Certificate Program for concurrent and post-graduate students. Bethanie is currently the Middle Tennessee Coordinator for UT's Human-Animal Bond in Tennessee (HABIT) program where she helps offer animal assisted interventions to victims of violence, abuse, and neglect.

Human-Animal Bond in Tennessee (HABIT) is a volunteer-based animal assisted intervention program sponsored by the University of Tennessee (UT) College of Veterinary Medicine. Started in 1986 by veterinarian Dr. John New, HABIT coordinates volunteers with medically and behaviorally screened dogs, cats, and rabbits with agencies that want visits from therapy animals. HABIT volunteer teams routinely visit hospitals, schools, courts, assisted living facilities, and many other types of agencies; we even have volunteers who visit accountants during tax season! As of this writing, HABIT has over 600 volunteer handler-animal teams and approximately 300 facilities that receive HABIT visits.

While HABIT thrived since its creation, it had been limited to East Tennessee. That changed in 2018 when the Tennessee Office of Criminal Justice Programs (OJCP) approached HABIT with an interesting proposition. OCJP wanted to bring the potential benefits of animal-assisted interventions into agencies that serve victims of crime, specifically survivors of domestic violence, child abuse, and elder abuse in Middle Tennessee. To accomplish this goal, a Middle Tennessee HABIT coordinator position was created, funded through the Crime Victim's Fund established by the Victims of Crime Act.

It turned out that I was uniquely qualified for this job which requires knowledge of not only animal assisted interventions but also victims' related services. I earned my master's and PhD at the University of Tennessee with a focus in veterinary social work. Veterinary social work is a specialized area of social work practice that branches into four general practice areas: animal related grief and bereavement; animal-assisted interventions; compassion fatigue and conflict management; and the Link between human and animal violence, which became my area of expertise. At this point in my career, I had experience working in child welfare and domestic violence, including employment with a statewide coalition, which meant I have a good working knowledge of the victim services agencies available. Conveniently, I was also living in the geographic area targeted by the grant and was able to hit the ground running.

As the Middle Tennessee HABIT Coordinator, I am responsible for the day-to-day development and administration of the program in that part of the state, which means I don't have "typical days". Recruitment of volunteers with suitable animals as well as agencies who would like to have HABIT volunteers visit has been my greatest priority. I regularly host information meetings for potential volunteers and agency representatives, table local events, attend professional meetings, and speak at conferences. Evening or weekend events are common so people who work during the day are able to attend, leading me to flex my time. Comfortable weather is needed for local pet-related outdoor events so late spring and early fall are particularly busy.

Once I have recruited new volunteers, I observe their animal evaluations and, assuming they pass, their first visits. I spend quite a bit of time driving, mostly around Nashville and the surrounding counties. Then, there's the paperwork. The HABIT program itself requires several forms including volunteer applications, behavior profiles, medical forms, registry check, and forms acknowledging duties as mandatory reporters of abuse as a way of documenting suitability and allowing the volunteers to be covered by our liability insurance. Meeting state and federal grant funding requirements entails a great deal more, and I am responsible for our data management and meeting quarterly reporting deadlines.

Growth of HABIT in Middle Tennessee has been steady, but slow. While HABIT has the advantage of name recognition in East Tennessee due to its longevity and good reputation, that is not the case in this region of the state. Networking, marketing, and publicity are a much larger portion of my job than I anticipated. Additionally, while most victim service agencies recognize the potential benefit of having therapy animal visits, many find the idea of adding another project on to an already full plate to be overwhelming. Bringing agencies on board often involves several meetings with different levels of agency staff and administration and a lot of back and forth communication to make sure the program is implemented as smoothly as possible. Communication skills, both oral and written, are absolutely crucial in this position as well as comfort with public speaking.

While the HABIT program has been in Middle Tennessee for a relatively short period of time, we can already see the impact we're making. Our HABIT teams have helped a client come out of a panic attack which let them continue talking to an advocate; listened to the child of a homicide victim talk about her "mommy who is in heaven;" and calmed angry teen-aged boys living in residential group homes. Our HABIT dogs' ears have soaked up the tears of people who are having the worst day of their lives and helped them move forward with a smile.

To practice ethically and to advance the field, we need practitioners who are educated in evidence-based AAI practices and who can contribute to that evidence base through research. UT Veterinary Social Work (vetsocial-work.utk.edu) started the first veterinary social work certificate program, and other universities are developing programs like it. It is my hope that as the field becomes more recognized, AAI programs will be considered an essential part of a well-rounded, trauma-informed approach to working with people.

24 A Social Worker's Experience at a Veterinary School and Teaching Hospital

Eric Richman

Eric Richman, MSW, LICSW, is a clinical social worker at Cummings Veterinary Medical Center at Tufts University. He provides counseling and support services to clients and staff at both the small and large animal hospitals. Eric provides support during emergencies, counsels clients who are caring for sick or dying animals, and offers equine-assisted learning for veterinary students and staff.

I transitioned into the field of veterinary social work after a 25-year career working at large teaching hospitals in and around Boston, Massachusetts. My previous work experience was in substance abuse and psychiatric treatment, followed by medical social work, primarily working within a liver and kidney transplant program. Teaching hospitals afforded me the opportunity to work in an interdisciplinary environment where people from various disciples would collaborate to best serve a patient's unique needs.

Organ transplantation is a fascinating field that has both lifesaving success, as well as its fair share of tragic losses. Working in this setting helped hone my skills in helping people struggle with difficult decisions and end of life care and support. In some ways, veterinary social work has similar challenges in terms of helping clients who have animals with acute or chronic health issues.

Starting around 2010, veterinary teaching hospitals began to employ social workers and other mental health professionals on a more consistent basis. The role of a social worker at a veterinary school teaching hospital can be narrow in scope, focusing primarily on the emotional needs of clients bringing in acute or chronically ill animals for treatment and grief counseling. However, in my role at a veterinary teaching hospital, the use of social work-related skills has been expansive. This is in part due to the nature of social work training as well as the openness of my university to utilize social work skills in a variety of settings.

In addition to direct client counseling around medical decision making for a sick animal, my role involves grief counseling with adults and children. This role is very important in a society that often devalues or ignores the role of pet loss and the impact it has on individuals and families. Part of a social worker's role in this setting is to validate the loss of an animal in someone's life and recognize the importance of the human-animal bond.

Having the experience and skills of developing support groups for patients in a medical setting struggling with liver and kidney disease or recovering from transplant surgery, it was a logical step for me to establish support groups in a veterinary setting. Specifically, pet loss groups allow individuals to share their grief in a setting where others can understand and provide mutual support in a safe and nonjudgmental setting.

At some veterinary teaching hospitals, the role of a social worker can also include the opportunity to work in a teaching role, lecturing to veterinary students as part of a larger course on the human-animal relationship. This teaching focuses on helping veterinary students understand grief and loss as it relates to interactions they will have with clients once they leave the classroom and enter the clinical setting. Additionally, it is an opportune time to help students begin to explore their own grief history and how they view loss and death in their own lives. In better understanding their own history and reaction to loss, they will be more equipped at helping clients faced with end of life care and decisions about their companion animals.

Perhaps one of the most exciting opportunities for social workers at some veterinary teaching hospitals has been in the area of equine-assisted learning (EAL) to help both students and veterinary staff address a number of important school and workplace challenges. EAL is an experiential learning method with horses that focuses on learning from doing various interactive activities with horses. The activity is followed by a facilitated debriefing session to help individuals make parallels from what they learned within their session and their own day-to day environment. Examples include topics such as self-awareness, team interactions, leadership roles, and communication skill development.

The benefits of EAL also extend to the horses. At our hospital, we use teaching horses that help students learn important equine skills and medical procedures. The horses appear to enjoy many of the activities during an EAL session, providing stimulation and enrichment, as well as a break from the clinic environment. This is a wonderful example of a mutually beneficial human-animal interaction.

Our satellite community clinic, which provides low cost veterinary services to underserved communities, presents another opportunity for social work involvement. In collaboration with the clinic Medical Director, we developed a program to imbed a master's level social work intern into the clinic to offer services to pet owners visiting the community clinic. The intern has the opportunity to practice assessments and interventions, and develop and implement core social work skills and competencies related to cultural humility and knowledge of social, economic, and environmental inequities.

Based on my experience in a veterinary school and teaching hospital, social workers and other social and behavioral professionals have a great deal to offer clients, students, faculty, house officers, and staff. As outlined above, our unique skill set can be used in a variety of settings and interactions to positively contribute to the veterinary profession and the development of future veterinary professionals.

25 Supporting Students and Companion Animals in University and Community Settings

Clarissa Uttley

Clarissa Uttley, PhD, is a professor of education at Plymouth State University in New Hampshire. Her teaching focuses on graduate level research design and assessment courses and undergraduate human-animal interaction special programming. In addition to coordinating the on-campus pet therapy program, she also supports the regional restorative justice program through consultation and individual case referrals. She develops professional development opportunities for pet therapy animal handlers specifically focusing on assessing the level of engagement and enjoyment the therapy animal is experiencing during the visits.

My interest in the field of human-animal interaction began before I did. My parents had companion animals when I was born and my 'siblings' were a dachshund named Schnappsee and three Pekin ducks. In fact, I really don't have photos of me with my parents for the first six months of my life—all the photos are of me with the critters! Growing up with companion animals and having parents who exposed me to animals of all sorts served as a strong foundation for my love and appreciation of animals.

After high school, moving out, and adopting my own first pet (a Maine coon named Clio), I became the Education Specialist for a small zoo. This position offered me opportunities to work with common and exotic animals, develop educational curriculum, and define my personal philosophy on how humans should interact with non-human animals.

Through my work at the zoo, I meet people with limited exposure to animals, who never contemplated that animals benefitted humans in ways other than as a food source, and others who had thought deeply about what it meant to care for animals. Each experience helped me think about messages people receive about the impact of animals on human lives. I started to read scientific articles and professional journals to keep informed of how science was addressing these issues.

One of the pieces I read was a short satire article printed in a zoological journal. This article, written from a dog's perspective, focused on feelings the dog had when people would try to pet his head. The 'author' discussed feeling violated, demeaned, and under the authority and power of those who pat his head. I would never forget this article. I read the article in the mid-1990s and the message it sent has left a tremendous impact on my work with both humans and non-humans. I left my work at the zoo and decided to pursue a higher education degree in early childhood studies. I wanted to explore how children developed concepts of and respect for animals. How we show respect and ask permission to engage with others is central to my work with children, therapy animals, and their handlers. My education continued from an associate's degree in early childhood through a PhD in psychology and a career in higher education as a professor in an education department.

As faculty, I engage in service activities to the university and our surrounding community. Many of my service commitments involve working with pet therapy teams on campus and with vulnerable populations in the region. Students have embraced our 'Dorm Dogs' (the name of our on-campus program during its first two years) and 'Building Dogs' (its current name) and their handlers through weekly, scheduled visits to specific buildings, at specific times each week and extra visits during more stressful times of the year. One challenge with my job is educating people who have not had experience with establishing pet therapy programs in college/university settings. These programs are very different from traditional college programs due to potential liability issues and federal regulations. Creating university-wide policy and ensuring that everyone adheres to those policies can be challenging. Monitoring the visits in addition to conducting my normal work responsibilities can also be a challenge. Visits last one hour, but I dedicate more time to ensure that therapy teams are comfortable and safe in their setting. Above all else, I want to confirm that our therapy program maintains safety for all involved.

It is in these visits that I get to see the benefits companion animals bring to the lives of so many individuals. Therapy teams originally expected the dogs would relieve student stress, but I don't think they realized how much they would influence the culture of the entire campus. Faculty and staff join students in visiting the therapy teams and talk about everyday activities outside of the classroom, without any pressure of the student-professor relationship. Everyone engaging in the campus pet therapy program is just people who enjoy being around animals! Hearing faculty or students say 'This made my day' or 'You don't know how bad I needed this visit today' is the best part of my job!

The beauty, and struggle, with my job is that I carved out this role for myself based on my personal experiences and my academic training. The university did not hire me for this specific role. Sadly, the role of Campus Pet Therapy Program Coordinator would not likely exist if I were to leave my position as a faculty member. As the driving force behind this program, I needed to gather evidence that this type of program was included in other universities, that there was potential benefit to the campus community, and that the pet therapy teams were properly certified. Curating the right type and amount of evidence is an ever-changing challenge as university and federal policies change.

A main resource when developing the on-campus pet therapy program was the Pet Partners website (petpartners.org) and Phil Arkow's guidebook, published by the Latham Foundation, *How to Start a "Pet Therapy" Program* (www.latham.org/Issues/Pet_Therapy.pdf). In addition, I reviewed university housing policies, the Americans with Disabilities Act, and other federal policies that might influence university policies and practices. Staying abreast of legal issues affecting on-campus pet therapy programs was a new area for me and I learned a great deal about blending respect for regulatory bodies and passion for a field I know helps so many people, especially stressed out college students!

This work takes a great deal of collaboration from many stakeholders (campus administration, faculty, students, pet therapy teams, etc.) in order to remain effective. However, once all the pieces are in place the results are meaningful to all involved and provide me with a great sense of accomplishment and purpose.

26 "Yes, I Work With Animals . . . No, I'm Not a Vet"—Animal–Assisted Intervention and the Indian Experience

Georgitta Valiyamattam

Georgitta Valiyamattam is an assistant professor in the Department of Applied Psychology at GITAM University, Visakhapatnam, India. Prior to this position, she worked as a Fulbright-Nehru Doctoral scholar at the Centre for the Human Animal Bond at the University of Purdue. Georgitta also partners with the Visakha Society for the Protection and Care of Animals (VSPCA)—a local animal welfare organization involved in regulating and scaling up their AAI programs along with other broader interests in animal welfare.

My journey into the field of animal-assisted intervention (AAI) was largely unplanned. Various positive experiences with animals since childhood had made me passionate about the animal world. However, I had little knowledge that this could also become a professional pursuit. While exploring options to pursue doctoral research in developmental disabilities, I chanced upon Dr. O'Haire's article reviewing the benefits of AAI for children with autism (O'Haire, 2013). This was in 2013, and a whole new world opened up for me. Having convinced my mentors in India of the research I wished to undertake (with no prior expertise, they were highly sceptical), I plotted out my own journey—reading extensive amounts of literature and completing an advanced certification in AAI offered by the University of North Texas under the mentorship of Dr. Cynthia Chandler. To gain broader expertise in the field, both in terms of research and practise, I applied for a Fulbright grant that enabled me to be a visiting scholar at the Center for the Human-Animal Bond at Purdue under Drs. Alan Beck and Marguerite O'Haire. Subsequently, I returned to India to complete my dissertation in which I examined, using an eye tracking paradigm, the social facilitation effects of animals for children with autism.

My work in the field, both as a doctoral student and later as a professional, has spanned both academia and practice. My average work-week is divided between teaching, research and practise. My practise involves biweekly visits to two special education schools for children with developmental disabilities. I conduct individually modified animal-assisted activity (AAA) sessions with guinea pigs, working with children on skills related to feeding, grooming and playing with the animals. While my University does not have a human–animal interaction (HAI) related course, I try and incorporate HAI principles within the content of the other courses that I teach (i.e., Lifespan Development and Positive Psychology). I am also involved with research examining how animals may impact visual attention and social functioning in children with autism.

Much of the AAI work that I do is voluntary and unpaid, yet comes with benefits that include recognition and positions on institutional and advisory panels by virtue of being an AAI professional. A foremost challenge that I have faced as an AAI professional in India revolves around explaining what I do. People often assume that I am a veterinarian and do not comprehend the difference between medically treating animals versus incorporating animals in psychological treatment processes. Convincing institutions of the benefits of AAI is also challenging, given that their conceptualizations of animals often orbit around rigid notions of harm or infections from animal contact. Patience is the key in such circumstances. To counter these limitations, I often offer to organize a small demonstration of AAI for teachers and caregivers and this is usually very effective.

I find that the most rewarding part of AAI work is seeing how children with developmental disabilities enjoy the presence of animals. Knowing that they often recognize me because of my animal co-workers is endearing and the instances of small yet significant improvements made due to the presence of animals in the therapeutic context are gratifying. It is also heartening to see how curious and receptive students are whenever I incorporate elements of HAI into their coursework; it gives me hope of a next generation of AAI professionals.

Over the next 5–10 years I see more positions opening up in academia and practice for an HAI professional and more research institutions collaborating on HAI research in India and other non-Euro American settings. Considering the growing pet market in these regions and the burgeoning enthusiasm that makes all things related to companion animals lucrative, the field also stands the risk of being misinterpreted and misused. Hence I would encourage those aiming for a career in HAI/AAI to be formally trained in the standards of the practice and to affiliate with organizations like the International Society for Anthrozoology (ISAZ) or the International Association of Human-Animal Interaction Organizations (IAHAIO) for a constructive connection with a global community of professionals. Ample AAI experience (hands-on and shadowing) within a local setting would be beneficial for a culturally relevant understanding of its nuances. Learning from the experiences of other professionals in related fields such as animal behaviour or welfare can also be helpful.

Being an HAI professional in India, one may also experience an inevitable overlap of roles with closely related fields such as animal welfare or ethics. As this may seem overwhelming at times, it is important to assess what particular field is the best fit for you. While charting out my career in HAI had its share of sacrifices and discouragements, I find, in retrospect, the journey to have been enormously rewarding. I therefore definitely encourage a career path in human-animal interaction for those interested in this line of work. As in any emerging field, there will certainly be a sizeable share of trials, but I believe that the strength of biophilia and the beauty of its manifestations are sufficiently invigorating. One of my favourite memories is of a largely non-verbal child with autism who after an AAI session asked through monosyllables and gestures if he could carry Sophie, my guinea pig co-therapist, back home with him. Moments like this are what keep me motivated and engaged.

Reference

O'Haire, M. E. (2013). Animal-assisted intervention for autism spectrum disorder: A systematic literature review. *Journal of Autism and Developmental Disorders, 43*(7), 1606–1622. doi:10.1007/s10803-012-1707-5. PMID: 23124442

Part III

For Profit, Not For Profit and Government

27 Making a Difference as an Animal–Assisted Interactions Program Coordinator

Tanya K. Bailey

Tanya K. Bailey, MSW, LICSW, is the Animal-Assisted Interactions Program Coordinator at the University of Minnesota (UMN). She directed one of the first therapeutic farms in the Twin Cities and teaches several graduate courses in AAI at UMN. In 2013, she established UMN's Pet Away Worry and Stress (PAWS) program, the first university-based, multi-species AAI program offered year-round for student mental health.

I encountered the constructs of "animal-assisted therapy" (AAT) and the "human-animal bond" (HAB) in the 1990s during my graduate studies in social work. Because there were so few people exploring ways animals impacted human mental health, I was afforded a unique opportunity to be part of a time of rich development, collaboration, and mentoring. However, I also experienced a high level of skepticism and confusion when I first started my studies in AAI, frequently hearing that my career path existed in veterinary medicine, not human health and well-being. Despite a lack of recognition that the natural world was a system of influence for healthy human development, my professors supported my determined pursuit of HAB inquiry.

Shortly after receiving my master's degree in social work, I attended a seminar by a distinguished founder of the AAT field, Dr. R. K. Anderson. Dr. Anderson's guidance throughout my career gave me confidence to pursue my path in AAI which has included starting one of the first nonprofit therapeutic farms in the Twin Cities (Minneapolis/Saint Paul, Minnesota, USA) for at-risk youth and families, developing some of the first activity manuals for therapists and educators, training others on canine- and equine-specific AAI program models, and serving on national AAI boards that created standards and practices which continue to guide the field today.

In 2012, I was recruited to join the University of Minnesota (UMN) as the Animal-Assisted Interactions Program Coordinator. In this role, I developed and taught three graduate courses in AAI and partnered with a wide variety of animals to provide AAI programming with community partners. One of these groups included UMN students and in the fall of 2013, I implemented a pilot AAI program at Boynton Health called PAWS—Pet Away Worry and Stress. Initially, PAWS met weekly for two hours throughout the academic year. Seven years later, PAWS has grown to four days a week plus monthly evening and summer sessions throughout the academic year. PAWS receives over 11,000 visits from students annually and includes over 120 registered therapy animal teams that have involved dogs, cats, rabbits, miniature horses, guinea pigs, fancy rats, llamas, and chickens. Furthermore, I am the Principal Investigator for a multi-year study examining how PAWS impacts college student stress and mental health.

An average day at work for me primarily consists of program oversight and implementation. Because PAWS operates in eight different locations, I must anticipate and organize varying logistics for each two-hour session. I am also one of at least five to six therapy animal teams at each session which allows me to keep a pulse on the wide variety of human-animal interactions as well as monitor student emotions and behaviors should additional mental health support be needed. The remaining parts of each day include some combination of team recruitment, orientation and training, program research and evaluation, presentations, and planning for future AAI endeavors.

I find the three most rewarding aspects of PAWS to be: 1) engaging with students—I get to know many students and they openly share their struggles as well as how much the animals matter to them; for some, PAWS has literally saved their lives; 2) working with the AAI teams—it is because of these open-hearted and dedicated AAI teams that PAWS has grown into the success it is today; and 3) sharing this work with health promotion colleagues who are highly dedicated to college student health and social justice—I constantly learn from and am inspired by them every day. In contrast, the most challenging part of my job is the recognition that college mental health is a product of so many systemic influences. While I cannot change the difficult realities so many students face, my lived HAB experiences give me confidence in knowing that even one interaction with an animal can provide comfort, a safe place, and hope.

I attribute part of my success in AAI to three aspects: 1) obtaining a degree in a viable professional field and gaining extensive experience with many groups of people and in many unique mental health settings; 2) devoting significant time to learn about, train, and practice with various multi-species partners; and 3) learning ways to effectively develop AAI programs and facilitate group process. In addition, I also suggest a few more ways to bolster your AAI aptitude and skill. Know the history of this field—it is imperative that you have a foundation, context, and appreciation of the progress education and healthcare has made by including animals in programs and services compared to even a few short years ago. Rely on others for help—you do not have to take on the immense effort required to start your own AAI nonprofit or consulting service. Instead, I recommend working within an agency or business to provide your AAI services because their established operational infrastructure and collegial support will help sustain you through this hard work. Be a critical thinker and conscientious consumer—the approaches, frameworks, and beliefs in the AAI field vary greatly and false or misleading information conveyed in classes, workshops, and research articles can cloud an accurate portrayal of current state. I continue to learn by reading the professional journals *Animals & Society*, *Anthrozoös*, *Human-Animal Interaction Bulletin*, and *People & Animals*; and attending/presenting at the national and international conferences and events listed by the International Society of Anthrozoölgy (ISAZ) and the International Association of Human-Animal Interaction Organizations (IAHAIO). And finally, embrace the exciting proposition that a lifetime of owning animals, a weekend workshop, or a few college classes are only the beginnings of your AAI journey—a life-long avocation filled with countless hours of experiences on your way to mastery.

28 Changing Lives, One Service Dog at a Time

Sarah (Birman) Leighton

Sarah Leighton is the National Director of Training and Client Services with Canine Companions for Independence. In her current position, Sarah oversees the professional training and client services departments, working closely with fellow staff on program quality and advocacy efforts for service dog users both at home and abroad.

I was 5 years old when I first started campaigning for a dog from my parents. Over a decade-long crusade, I applied every ounce of my creativity. I tried: fact-based arguments (many people think Polaris, the North Star, is the brightest star in the sky; but did you know it is really Sirius, the dog star?); a marketing campaign (photos of golden retrievers, everywhere—behind the ketchup, on the mirror, in their shoes . . .); the "door in the face" technique (I can't have a pony? How about just a dog?); tantrums (ineffective); demonstrations of responsibility (volunteering for our local SPCA, walking the neighbor's dog); and many, many other bids over the years.

In spite of my efforts, I had limited success swaying my parents—until I turned 15, and into my life bounded a little golden retriever puppy by the name of Biscuit. Over the ten years of her life, Biscuit taught me first-hand the incredible value of the human-canine bond. With her by my side, I laughed more readily and connected with other people with ease. She was my steady friend through some of the most trying moments of my life. So, when, as a senior in college, a career counselor asked me what brought me the greatest joy, my answer was immediate: time with my dog and volunteering at the SPCA.

Truthfully, I hadn't considered work with dogs as a possible career. It seems absurd, in hindsight, but my focus at that time was on cognitive science, an emerging field that I found utterly fascinating. And yet, the reality of what constitutes a research position was not for me. I needed direct connection with people, to see the results of my work impacting the world in a more tangible way. Thankfully, the career counselor—to whom I owe a debt of gratitude—was able to connect the dots for me. As it turned out, my educational background in psychology and animal science, my direct experience with dogs, and even the customer service skills I had gained through summer jobs catering, all provided me with the well-rounded experience necessary to start a career as a service dog instructor.

There are many types of service dogs in the world; Canine Companions specifically trains dogs to assist their handler with a disability with tasks such as picking up dropped items, pulling a manual wheelchair, and turning lights on and off. Our dogs are trained to alert a person who is d/Deaf to important sounds, provide calming pressure to a child with autism, or wake a veteran with post-traumatic stress disorder from a nightmare—and so much more.

I absolutely loved my work as an instructor, so much so that I missed it on my days off. As an instructor, my job included not only training the dogs—smart, playful retriever breeds—in over 40 commands, but also ensuring they were comfortable around adaptive equipment and in many different environments. I provided demonstrations for campus visitors, worked with volunteer puppy raisers, and mentored apprentice instructors. I worked directly with our clients, conducting interviews with applicants and follow-up support for graduates, traveling to other states to meet with them in their communities. Best of all, I got to teach Team Training, a two-week class where students are matched with their new canine partner and learn to work together.

Since my promotion in 2016, I no longer work as closely with our clients, but the work is no less meaningful. As a member of the executive leadership team, I direct our training and client services department, working closely with our staff and board of directors to elevate our program as one of the most innovative and best respected in the world. I participate on committees with our accrediting organization, Assistance Dogs International, and am an active advocate for service dog users worldwide.

I consider myself truly lucky to have landed my dream job; most days this job doesn't even feel like work. Of course, there are challenges: dog training can be repetitive and physically tiring work, and all accredited service dog organizations are non-profits, meaning that pay is typically lower than it is in the for-profit sector (although great benefits can often help offset this significantly). For me, these challenges pale in comparison to the rewards: Every day I get to collaborate with other staff and volunteers who share my passion, and bear witness to the power of the human-canine connection to change lives. Service dogs give their handlers the gift of greater independence, and it's an honor to be a part of that journey.

Those interested in a career as a service dog instructor should consider education and experience in the following areas: animal science, psychology, education, and, of course, work with individuals with disabilities. It's important to develop comfort both working directly with animals, and with people, including public speaking. To learn more about this job, I encourage you to look into service dog schools in your area and sign up for a tour or consider volunteering as a puppy raiser. This type of volunteering will not only give you direct experience with the incredible mission of these organizations, it has the potential to profoundly change somebody's life. What greater gift can there be?

29 Canine–Assisted Family Treatment Court Coordinator

Megan Bridges

Megan Bridges, MS, AADC, is the Coordinator for the Calhoun County Family Drug Court, working with individuals with substance use disorders. She has trained two of her own dogs to assist her clients in the family drug court she coordinates. Megan also educates the public and professionals about the therapeutic benefits that animals can offer to those involved in the court system, as well as to providers, children, and the general public.

———————

A strong passion for helping others has been a part of my personality for as long as I can remember, though my vision and understanding of how to go about helping others has changed dramatically over the years. I dedicated my life to the field of substance abuse counseling and learning, and while I am confident and competent in my area of expertise, I firmly believe that there will never be an end to the knowledge and understanding I can gain and it is my responsibility to pursue that professional knowledge.

My passion for including animals in my work also started early in my life. As many young animal enthusiasts, my first career aspirations were to become a veterinarian or farmer. My parents pushed me to go to college where I developed an interest in working animals such as police horses, detection dogs, and therapy dogs. At that time I was unsure how I would be able to include animals in my career, but I knew that I would.

I completed a bachelor's degree with a double major in criminal justice and psychology. The psychology degree afforded me many opportunities to work with animals because the primary focus was on behavior analysis. I was able to complete labs in which I trained pigeons and an internship where I was able to learn the basics of training bomb detection dogs. After completing the bachelor's degree, I completed a master's program for criminal justice, and one for counselor education. Through my studies and self-reflection, I began to realize that I was not interested in pursuing a career in criminal justice so I began my career as a counselor. Initially I was a counselor in a program for severely mentally ill people where I met an exceptional mentor. He taught me what it meant to be a competent professional. Through some shifting of positons in the company, I landed in a position that offered me the opportunity to become a certified substance abuse counselor, and finally the coordinator of the Calhoun County Family Drug Court, a family reunification court that focuses on the substance abuse treatment needs of parents who are also involved in the child protective services system. In this position, no two days are exactly the same. There is enough variability that it keeps me interested, and just enough routine to keep me comfortable. Most days I interact with clients for 5–45 minutes at a time, either in brief counseling sessions or in treatment team meetings. My canine partner for the day, Whisper (a papillon) or Squiggle (a mutt), typically accompanies me to those sessions and meetings.

The most rewarding part of my job is seeing my clients and my canine partner form genuine connections that lead to healthy behavior changes in the client's life. One of the most memorable moments was when I was visiting the child welfare office and two young children emerged from an office and my partner, Whisper, dragged me to meet the boys. When I approached the boys, they smiled and knelt down to pet Whisper, who was excited to see them. I began to explain that Whisper works with me in my office and is allowed to visit the child welfare office from time to time. The children looked up at me as they were petting Whisper and said, "Oh, we know. We met him last time we were here." The kids remembered Whisper and he remembered them even though I had not. They had made a meaningful enough connection from the first time they met that all three of them had positive memories of each other.

My job is challenging in general—working with individuals who struggle with making good decisions and are not healthy enough at times to address their poor decisions—can be difficult. However in terms of including human-animal interaction in this work, challenges also include educating others about the differences in therapy, service, emotional support, facility dogs, and other working animals. While I have found most people to be receptive to the information I am able to provide, I do still see some people who are resistant to accepting the benefits of human-animal interaction in the healthcare and legal systems.

If I could give one piece of advice to people interested in becoming a partner with a working animal or including human-animal interaction into their work, I would say become competent! Attend training, network with other professionals, look outside of your specific field, and gather as much knowledge as possible. Never stop learning.

One of my favorite places to go for information is the International Institute for Animal Assisted Play Therapy®. Dr. Rise VanFleet and Traci Faa-Thompson have done an exceptional job gathering, organizing, and producing accessible information regarding the partnering with animals in therapeutic interventions. Their book, *Animal Assisted Play Therapy*

(2017), is a must-have for anyone interested in the field of animal assisted therapy.

Reference

VanFleet, R., & Faa-Thompson, T. (2017). *Animal assisted play therapy*. Sarasota, FL: Professional Resource Press.

30 Nurse-Led Canine-Assisted Intervention Practice

Cindy Brosig

Cindy Brosig has an MS in nursing with an emphasis in Animal-Assisted Therapy. She created Operation H.E.E.L., the first nurse-led Animal-Assisted Intervention practice fostering the health benefits of the human-animal bond. Cindy also instructs a Therapy Dog Prep Class and is an evaluator for canine skills testing.

———————

Canine-Assisted Interventions (CAI) in the health care setting was created and formally implemented in 1976 by Elaine Smith, a registered nurse and the Founder of Therapy Dogs International, the first Therapy Dog organization established in the United States. As a nurse working in the community health care setting, it was a natural progression for me to establish the first nurse-led Animal-Assisted Intervention (AAI) practice for children and adults based on current research supporting the healing qualities of the human animal bond. Witnessing the lives changed by working with a dog moved me to provide an essential health service for the community that is dedicated to the prevention, maintenance, and recovery of human dis-ease through the presence of dogs.

My interest in the field began with my faithful canine companion, Aggie, a mixed-breed dog rescued at approximately 2 years of age, reportedly running alone on a rural, dusty farm road in Indiana. Not only had I noticed Aggie's patience with young children as she gently maneuvered herself around them so they could touch her soft coat, but she also caught the eye of special education teachers who invited her to visit with disabled children while waiting for the arrival of their school buses. Every day we witnessed the pure joy Aggie brought to these otherwise quiet, seemingly unresponsive students their squeals of excitement and uncontrolled, yet thoughtful movements of their arms and legs. It was then that I knew that dogs offered something special to humans facing physical, mental, and circumstantial challenges, and I decided to devote my graduate studies in nursing to prove this.

Through my research of utilizing AAI in patient care I found that it is not enough to have a thorough understanding of human dis-ease and human interaction with another species. Researching, practicing, and applying knowledge of canine behavior and health is another important component to consider that not only helps to nurture the beneficial, healing relationship between humans and dogs but also protects the health and wellness of the canine companion. For this reason, I continue to collaborate with my sister, USAF Major Nancy Lester, a veterinarian with a master's degree in public health, take dog-training classes, complete canine skills testing, and work privately with dog trainers. I attribute my knowledge of canine welfare and behavior through raising and training my second adopted dog, Ted, a 6-year-old mixed breed rescue who completed his Canine Good Citizen Test and registration as a nationally recognized Therapy Dog at only 1 1/2 years old, quite remarkable for a dog his age.

After several years of volunteering as a registered Therapy Dog team for U.S. military members, U.S. veterans, and their family members Ted and I honed our skills in meeting the physiological, social, and emotional needs of humans. Concurrently, I dedicated my graduate studies in nursing on evidenced-based practices that focused on AAI for different patient populations. Certificate programs and continuing education credits in AAI are available through online platforms, but they usually only cover usage of basic terminology with minimal understanding of canine behavior, not actual therapeutic approaches.

Challenges in my work include using the term "pet therapy" for both informal, therapeutic visits and measurable, goal-based therapy sessions. This causes confusion in differentiating types of services sought by individuals. Additionally, clients are more familiar with nurses providing traditional medical care in an institution, not for their ability to use innovative, therapeutic interventions in private practice.

The gift of being present during the subtle moments of transformation and understanding between a child and a dog is revered. Knowing these interactions will positively affect the quality of life for that individual continues to inspire my work advocating for AAI as an evidenced-based tool to be used to achieve health and wellness. Working with dogs decreases the use of medications (and in many cases individuals cease to use medications), enhances relationships with family and friends, and reminds us of what it means to have compassion for others and for oneself.

For AAI to be successful, the working dog must have the freedom to interact naturally, in play and at rest. It is also crucial to take time in developing the human-animal bond, adjusting for potential personality conflicts (e.g., a dog that is too happy can be over-stimulating for a child experiencing symptoms of depression), and taking time for closure at the end of the therapeutic relationship. I foster an individual's independence working with a dog, not dependence working with a dog.

I began this career path thinking I needed to train a dog to be therapeutic. While basic obedience skills are necessary to safely maneuver in public, dogs are sentient beings; many sense when they are needed for support. I strongly encourage anyone entering this field to start by volunteering to care for rescue dogs to interpret stress, calming, and positive canine behaviors. In turn, you will be enriching a dog's life and learning a bit about yourself, too.

31 Promoting Animal Welfare in a Context of International Development

A Career in the Non-Governmental Sector

Ashleigh F. Brown

Ashleigh F. Brown is the Global Animal Welfare Advisor at Brooke, an equine welfare organisation. Ashleigh is also a lay advisor for the Royal College of Surgeons of Edinburgh where she is lay representative on the Research Committee, International Committee and Global Surgery Foundation, and for the Academy of Medical Royal Colleges in London. She is a member of TEDxLondon's management team.

From an early age I had great interest and compassion for all animals, and when I started riding lessons at the age of 10, my enduring love of horses was born! I completed an undergraduate degree in equine science, a qualification in teaching English to speakers of other languages, a master of science in animal behaviour and welfare, and accumulated years of practical experience with a variety of horses (and their owners) and other species (e.g., rescued sloth bears and domesticated elephants). All of those experiences, in combination with extensive international travel, were highly pertinent to my current roles as Global Animal Welfare Advisor at Brooke and as a trustee for two animal protection and conservation charities—Friends of Inti Wara Yassi which supports wildlife in the Bolivian Amazon, and the League Against Cruel Sports which protects animals in the United Kingdom.

Brooke is an international non-governmental organisation (NGO) improving the lives of working equine animals and the people who depend upon them, operational in South Asia, Sub-Saharan Africa, the Middle East and Central America. I joined in 2009, determined to make a difference to the world's neediest horses, donkeys and mules, and found my perfect role—I could contribute meaningfully to a cause I believed in whilst combining my scientific background, equestrian skills and passion for travel.

Keen to continue learning, I undertook further postgraduate qualifications in adult education and international development management, and now pursue several additional professional activities alongside my animal welfare interests. These include curating speakers and organising events as a member of the TEDxLondon team; supporting improvement in human healthcare as a lay advisor for the Royal College of Surgeons of Edinburgh and the Academy of Medical Royal Colleges in London; and mentoring students and young people. My wanderlust has not yet abated, and I have worked or travelled in more than 75 countries (so far).

My work at Brooke is varied, rewarding and busy! Essentially, I provide animal welfare, behaviour or equestrian expertise—whenever and wherever required—to ensure animal welfare is prioritised and reflected in organisational activities and operational standards. I develop indicators to measure animal welfare and human-animal interaction; identify and mitigate animal welfare risk in project or fund-raising activities; and support colleagues with appraisal of new project proposals. Building others' capabilities is an important part of my role, and I deliver training internationally in animal welfare, equine behaviour, welfare-friendly handling and welfare assessment, and create learning materials and opportunities to help others strengthen their knowledge and practical skills. I also contribute to profile- and fund-raising through representation at scientific conferences, speaking engagements and donor events; as deputy chair of the Animal Welfare and Ethical Review Body, I consider ethical implications for animals and humans involved in research and data collection.

As a charity trustee, my role is to provide guidance on strategy and policy, ensure the charities are well-governed and accountable, and that resources are utilised in accordance with their objectives and charitable remit.

Working at the intersection of animal welfare and international development has allowed me to gain an understanding of the role of human behaviour change in improving animal welfare. As working equids are intrinsic to the livelihoods of those who use them, the human-animal dyad is central to this work. In this and other scenarios, it is important to appreciate the context-specific motivating and inhibiting factors influencing people's treatment of animals, and aim to proactively engage with all stakeholders and, wherever possible, create participatory interventions to achieve positive change in animal welfare practices.

The animals are both the most rewarding and most challenging aspect of my work. Exposure to their suffering never gets easier, and even after many years I still find it deeply distressing; some horrifying visions can never be unseen. However, it is also these animals—their strength, courage, resilience and inherent goodness—who are my continual motivation to make the world a better place for them. It is very rewarding when, for example, community members in Pakistan are proud to show me how they are preventing heat stress in horses, or re-visiting garbage-collection donkeys in Senegal to see incredible improvement in their condition. There is also hope in reflecting upon how many animals' lives have been improved around the world as a result of effective work by NGOs, and in creating sustainable change that will benefit many more in the future.

How This Job Has Affected My Lifestyle

Often, working for a NGO is not just a job but a lifestyle choice! Working internationally and travelling frequently can limit opportunity to participate in social events, hobbies or aspects of family life. There may be a requirement to work in insecure or dangerous environments, and a risk of illness or injury when conducting field work in remote locations and resource-poor contexts (particularly when physically working with animals). However, willingness to sacrifice some everyday norms and comforts will undoubtedly reap myriad rewards in terms of priceless learning opportunities, valuable friendships and wonderful cultural experiences that would never otherwise be feasible, in addition to the satisfaction of contributing to a meaningful cause. To remain motivated and productive in the face of the inevitable challenges in this line of work, it is important to have a genuine passion for the cause.

Core Competencies and Skills Needed

Working in the NGO sector requires resilience, adaptability, patience and the confidence to be able to make decisions, respond to emergent challenges under pressure and provide guidance to others based on individual expertise and knowledge of good practice. It is also essential to be able to communicate effectively and respectfully with a wide variety of people from all walks of life, cultural backgrounds and differing perspectives. Having the self-awareness to reflect upon others' needs, expectations and contextual norms, and the ability to adapt language and behaviour according to the demographic of people you are interacting with is crucial to being able to work successfully and collaboratively with other stakeholders.

32 Advancing Standards and Professionalization in the Field of AAI

Taylor Chastain

Taylor Chastain, PhD, is the National Director of AAI Advancement for Pet Partners where she focuses on supporting research and professional development within the therapy animal arena. Taylor is also a dog trainer and Pet Partners team evaluator and has been a registered handler with Pet Partners since 2015.

Ever since rescuing my first pet in elementary school, my life has been filled with experiences that point to the power that animals have in the lives of humans. Early on, I considered a career in veterinary practice or animal science, but neither field seemed like a good fit given my desire to incorporate interactions with animals into the provision of human healthcare. When I first began discussing my specific goals as a freshman in college, advisors would often respond by telling me that the job that I wanted didn't yet exist. Nonetheless, they encouraged me to tailor my educational and vocational experiences in a way that would balance my knowledge and develop expertise related to both humans and animals.

I found that it was easiest to focus my educational efforts on learning about human mental health services. I completed my undergraduate degree in psychology, followed by my master's in mental health counseling. While I was in these programs, my vocational experiences were largely in the animal world. I volunteered with my therapy dogs and became a professional dog trainer. As I neared the end of my master's program, I was finally able to integrate my work with people and animals by incorporating my dogs into counseling sessions. My experiences in those sessions not only solidified my belief in the power of the human-animal connection, but they also inspired me to continue my education so that I would be optimally empowered to advocate for Animal Assisted Intervention (AAI). I went back to school to complete my doctorate in research psychology while investigating the intersection of pet ownership and domestic violence for the purposes of my dissertation project.

I am now enjoying my dream job at Pet Partners, one of the largest therapy animal organizations in the word. In my role as the National Director of

AAI Advancement, my primary objective is to motivate standardization and professionalization within the field. I work with researchers to design studies that are representative of best practices in AAI, and also help researchers with participant recruitment. I collaborate with a wide range of professionals from fields in which AAI are commonly incorporated, working together to identify gaps in education or applied practice that impact a practitioner's ability to effectively bring therapy animals into their work. An additional objective of my position is to raise awareness about therapy animal standards. I accomplish this by speaking and publishing materials for facilities, media outlets, and the general public to help empower consumers to engage in high-quality AAI. One of the greatest privileges of my jobs is that I'm able to connect with so many people who can relate to my passion for therapy animal work. Together, we see how the field is emerging, moving ever forward towards our goal of bringing the healing power of animals to as wide an audience as possible. While it can sometimes be overwhelming to know exactly where to focus our collaborative efforts, I am optimistic about the ways in which AAI is being developed and refined for the mutual benefit of the people and the animals who are involved in the intervention.

Even in the short amount of time that I have been out of school, I have witnessed a tremendous growth in the number of professionals who are also focusing on specializing in AAI as a major component of their vocational identity. When addressing people who aim to incorporate AAI into their work, I am inclined to pass along the same sage advice that I was given during my undergraduate experience: balance your career's development so that you are highly informed in your work with both humans and animals. Any time an animal is involved in a treatment plan, the practitioner must have the ability to understand the animal and thus advocate for its well-being. I would also suggest that people who are interested in this career become involved in the groups and networks of professionals with a shared interest in AAI. If there is a human-animal interaction interest group within your field's professional association, consider joining it. If no such group exists in your profession, perhaps you are just the person to step into a leadership role and create one. You might also find it beneficial to connect with AAI leaders who have different vocational focuses but who have led the way in their respected fields to establish standards within their discipline. Finally, stay active in your personal engagement with AAI. If you have a pet who is a candidate for therapy animal work, consider becoming registered with a reputable organization so that you can personally witness the impact of animal intervention. Advocates who do not have pets can also find opportunities to become engaged in AAI by shadowing visits, assisting with therapy animal evaluations, or looking into volunteer leadership roles within a therapy animal organization. By establishing your commitment to this field at all levels, you will be prepared to join in the movement to advance AAI and promote the continued recognition of the healing power of pets.

33 A Day in the Life of an Executive Director at an Animal Protection Think Tank

Ivy Collier

Ivy Collier is the Executive Director for the Animals and Society Institute where she is responsible for the mission, vision, strategy and fundraising efforts for the organization. Under Ivy's leadership the organization is focused on creating safer and more compassionate communities for all. Additionally, as an independent researcher, she studies animal ethics as well as animals and public policy.

———————

It was a dark, stormy night when my life was transformed. I wasn't planning on such a dramatic event, only a warm bowl of soup and watching my favorite TV show. But life had a different idea when I found a stray dog wandering in the rain. I stopped, put him in the car and took him home. He was a black chow-mix, very matted and thin. He was alone, soaking wet and afraid. I called my local animal shelter, and they advised me to search for the owner. I put up lost dog signs in the area and continued to contact the shelter to see if the owner called. Nobody called. I couldn't keep him as it was a violation to my lease and thus had no choice but to take him to the shelter. I'd never been inside a shelter before, and I was horrified. It was dark, damp and noisy. I was riddled with guilt, but the staff assured me they'd find him a loving home. But the truth is, they didn't, they euthanized him. They told me they simply did not have the space, that it was a hard decision to make, but one they must make on a regular basis. This was an eye-opening experience for me and led to my interest in learning about the plight of pet animals as well as farm animals and wildlife. I had found my calling—animal protection—and have never looked back.

I started volunteering with multiple animal shelters and activist groups. I completed my bachelor's degree in social psychology and then my master's degree in public affairs. Throughout my early career, I worked for conservation and animal welfare organizations, but I wanted a deeper understanding of the human-animal relationship. An internet search led me to the Animals & Society Institute (ASI), and I became a volunteer. A few years later I joined the ASI board, and in January of 2019 I became the Executive Director.

While my education helped prepare me for this position, my volunteer experience gave me hands-on knowledge needed to build the strong skillset necessary to work in the nonprofit world. As my career evolved, I learned that I needed specialized experience in nonprofit boards and fundraising. I sought out specific learning opportunities through professional Facebook groups, Joan Garry's blog, the Board Source and the Council of Nonprofits. I also joined the Association of Fundraising Professionals and took advantage of their continuing education opportunities. I subscribed to the Get Fully Funded program, an excellent source to learn new fundraising skills and planning, as well as the Chronicle of Philanthropy.

I am grateful that ASI is a leader in the human-animal interaction field and publishes two academic journals. I keep abreast of the field by reading these journals along with other research produced by Faunalytics. I subscribe to numerous HAI newsletters and Facebook pages and set up keyword alerts in Google and Academia.edu. Lastly, I connect with HAI professionals on LinkedIn. I recognize that keeping up with new research and nonprofit news can be overwhelming, so to help with this issue, I set a certain amount of time aside each day to scroll through alerts, newsletters and new information.

My position as Executive Director is to oversee the strategic plan, programs and governance for ASI. A few key responsibilities that I am responsible for include the organization budget, fundraising, marketing and community outreach. While my day-to-day activities are never the same, here's an example:

9:00am Quiet time. Review my to-do list. Read and reply to emails. Review donation list. Write thank you notes.
10:00 Make phone calls to donors, funders and vendors. Work on upcoming fundraising campaign strategy.
11:00 Meet with Board fundraising committee.
Noon Lunch.
1:00 Staff meeting.
2:00–4:00 Work on proposal draft for prospective foundation.
4:00–5:00 Prepare board report.
5:00–5:15 Review calendar and task list for tomorrow.

While ASI has standard office hours, donor meetings or phone conferences may warrant working evenings and weekends. Once or twice a week, I work additional hours in the evenings. The most rewarding part of my job is knowing that I am helping animals and people. When I turn on my computer each morning, I know that I am working to create a safer and more compassionate community for animals and people alike. I am lucky and blessed to work with the best team, individuals who share the same vision and are always ready to help and encourage each other to be the best they can be.

Human–animal studies (HAS) is a rapidly growing interdisciplinary field with a bright future. There are more HAS courses and majors than ever before. Countless HAS resources are being produced and are now interwoven throughout our society. My hope is that as the HAS field continues to evolve, it becomes more diverse in every sense; race, ethnicity, gender and thought. We have so much to learn from each other, the field will benefit from becoming as diverse and inclusive as possible.

The nonprofit sector has been growing over the past 30 years and is expected to continue to grow. I encourage anyone who wants a career that is rewarding and meaningful to strongly consider joining the nonprofit community.

34 Occupational Therapy

Using Meaningful Occupations to Enhance Function Throughout the Lifespan

Emily DeBreto

Emily DeBreto, MA, OTR/L, is a pediatric occupational therapist and certified brain injury specialist. She works with children and young adults who have complex medical conditions at Gillette Children's Specialty Healthcare in St. Paul, Minnesota. Emily developed the Animal-Assisted Therapy (AAT) program at Gillette and is working to expand the program to Gillette's outpatient pediatric clinics.

———————

I have always been driven to find a career that promotes function and quality of life. During my undergraduate coursework in psychology, I held volunteer and internship positions in healthcare and education, which later shaped my interest in the field of occupational therapy. One of the most formative experiences for me was the position I held as a personal care attendant. I worked with a child who had a genetic condition that affected her global development. My role was to help her gain independence in daily living, social, and leisure skills so that she could thrive in all of her natural environments. This experience opened my eyes to how I could positively impact someone's life in a meaningful way. After graduating with a degree in psychology, I had the opportunity to shadow and interview an occupational therapist (OT) in a pediatric hospital. I was inspired by the way the therapist skillfully used play exploration activities to improve the child's visual and fine motor skills. During the interview, I learned that a career in occupational therapy would allow me to combine my passion for working in healthcare with my background in psychology and my love for animals. These experiences are what led me to pursue a master's of arts degree in occupational therapy.

My current position as an occupational therapist is within a pediatric hospital that specializes in complex medical and genetic conditions. I evaluate and treat children and young adults on several inpatient units including: rehabilitation, neurosciences, intensive care, and orthopedic-surgical. As such, I work with patients recovering from elective surgeries, injuries, and acute illnesses. In an average day, I provide treatment to five to seven patients, complete medical documentation, attend family conferences, conduct evaluations, and collaborate with colleagues on the rehabilitation team. In addition to my role as therapist, I am the animal-assisted therapy (AAT) program lead. As program lead, I coordinate AAT sessions for physical, occupational, and speech therapists; conduct up-to-date literature reviews on AAT and human-animal interactions; revise and update clinical practice guidelines; and provide hands-on training and mentorship to both dog handlers and clinicians.

Playing an active role in an individual's recovery and observing the daily progress patients make are the two most rewarding and exhilarating aspects of my career. I am inspired when patients achieve their goals despite the new challenges they are facing. As appropriate to an individual's plan of care, I implement AAT in my practice to enrich the therapeutic environment and promote functional skills. My role during an AAT session is to facilitate goal-oriented skills while simultaneously collaborating with the dog handler in order to set the patient up for optimal participation in therapy. Skills that I promote during an AAT session may include: visual perception, active range of motion, functional mobility skills, fine motor skills, and/or executive functioning skills. I have witnessed a child move their arm for the very first time after a brain injury while reaching to brush, pet, feed, and play with the therapy dog. I have utilized therapy dogs during the occupation of play to promote visual scanning skills in children who have suffered a stroke as they search for hidden puzzle pieces buried under the dog's fur. Children who are generally anxious about moving or exploring their environment because of pain or anxiety demonstrate a calmer state simply by being in the presence of the animal. With these barriers removed, I am able to move their therapy goals forward, which is one of the greatest benefits of AAT. One of the biggest challenges with my career is witnessing the grief that patients and their loved ones face, especially when a full recovery is unlikely. Patients and families are coping with a change in function and a new reality, which can be both physically and emotionally devastating. Compassion fatigue exists in this field and reinforces the importance of self-care and work-life balance to avoid burnout.

Occupational therapy is a versatile and exciting career with excellent job security. Individuals who succeed in this profession are detail-oriented, compassionate, and have very strong interpersonal skills. As an occupational therapist, there are opportunities to work with people across the lifespan and in a multitude of settings. Occupational therapists in nursing homes, schools, and medical settings have the opportunity to use AAT in their practice. Additionally, occupational therapy is a wonderful avenue for utilizing and researching AAT. There are also opportunities within the OT profession to be involved in advocacy and healthcare legislation. Professional advancement is possible in this career but dependent upon each work setting. Program development, research, involvement in special projects, committee participation, and professional presentations are some of the ways a therapist can advance professionally. Occupational therapists also have the opportunity to assume leadership roles, including that of a rehab supervisor or manager.

I would encourage anyone interested in this field to pursue volunteer and/or job shadow experiences in healthcare, education, and/or community-based organizations. Interviewing an occupational therapist is an invaluable way to learn more about the nature and realities of the field. An excellent resource for learning about the field is the website for the American Occupational Therapy Association (www.aota.org). Another useful resource is the World Federation of Occupational Therapists webpage, found at www.wfot.org. Lastly, the American Journal of Occupational Therapy (AJOT) contains peer-reviewed journal articles on highly varied topic areas.

35 The Clinical Direction of Dogs

Matthew Decker

Matthew Decker is a US Marine veteran of the war in Iraq and the Executive Director of E5 Therapy, a mental health agency specializing in canine-assisted therapy for military veterans. He holds a license in clinical social work and has been working as an animal assisted therapist for ten years. He has assisted in building, developing, and supporting multiple service dog organizations in the Northern California region.

I unearthed my calling as a mental health provider while stationed in Iraq during Operation Iraqi Freedom. I found myself the unofficial platoon counselor assigned to help other warzone service members work through their mental health issues. "Anyone got a problem . . . see Decker!" was the solution to a variety of challenges, usually involving emotions and crying. After returning from deployment, I realized my calling and obtained my bachelor's degree in sociology from Arizona State. After some down–in–the–dirt clinical practice I went on to the University of Southern California for an MSW. As was my initial intention, in 2013 I joined the Veterans Administration (VA) as a medical and mental health social worker.

It was in 2010 while working in a community mental health clinic with at–risk kids that I discovered how dogs could enhance my practice. Another therapist brought her standard poodles to work and I noticed how this simple change affected the overall mood of the office. My natural childhood affinity for dogs kicked in, and I started reading more and more about human–canine connections. *How to Speak Dog* by Stanley Coren started me on a path that led to training my first therapy dog, Maggie. I started using the term "human-interaction therapy dog" to describe how Maggie worked with my clients. What occurred during these sessions was a special dog-client relationship, enhancing my work with these clients. Today, there is a burgeoning number of programs and professionals educating, training, and advising mental health teams on the practice of canine-assisted therapy.

A typical day for me starts with dog hugs, kisses, a trip to the gym, and then COFFEE. As the former Clinical Director of a service dog non-profit, I reviewed Veteran applications for service, translated mental health records into language a non-professional could understand, interviewed potential clients, facilitated connections with medical and mental health providers, and debriefed staff on the complex symptomatology that clients experience. Within the service dog agency, I ensured the entire staff used "best practices" in helping their Veteran clients succeed. In my position, I use canine-assisted therapy in two ways. First, I include dogs as part of the diagnostic, intervention, and overall treatment of clients. Second, I use canine therapy as "medication" in treating veterans for the symptoms of post-traumatic stress and other military-related mental health conditions.

Being the clinical director of a service dog agency requires hard work, long hours, a flexible schedule, and determination. The job may drain your energy, but will never leave you feeling empty. Most likely, you will be the only mental health subject-matter expert in your organization, which can be lonely and sometimes frustrating. Your teams will frequently not understand how you reach your client diagnoses. In time, the trainers and teams will grow to trust your direction and come to you for help.

So, what do you need to get started in this new profession? A master's degree in a mental health profession is required, and a license to practice mental health as an independent practitioner would also be helpful. Those are concurrent to acquiring significant training and skills with canine therapy. As a clinical director including canine therapy in your clinical work, it would be helpful to have gained previous experience with therapy dogs, trained a therapy dog, and provided canine-assisted therapy under the guidance of a professional canine therapist.

You can expect long hours and need a "whatever it takes" attitude to survive in this business. The fact is, no one schedules a crisis at a convenient time of day. These episodes occur at the most inconvenient moments—day and night, at all hours, and especially on the weekends (when you would rather be doing family outings). You will conduct crisis counseling, search for lost souls, look for their missing dogs, and support your training teams. As the Clinical Director, when your staff needs you—you go. Above all else, you must maintain unconditional positive regard for all parties involved. This is also one of the hardest values to teach your staff.

What do you get for all of this work? If you have the previous knowledge, skills, and experience listed, consider yourself a valuable commodity and important part of the organizational team. Most clinical director jobs are either within non-profit organizations, the VA, or Department of Defense. Nonprofit salaries are often lower than might be demanded by private, for-profit groups, but the salaries for government positions are often higher and more predictable than nonprofits. Most non-profit and private-sector clinics have yet to apply canine-assisted therapy to their work, but the field of canine-assisted therapy is growing. If this is what you want to do, it is important to find an organization willing to see canine-assisted therapy as an important tool in mental health treatment.

36 Animal Instincts

Following an Unmarked Path From Volunteerism to a Career in Human Animal Interaction

Marivic R. Dizon

Marivic R. Dizon, PhD, is Coordinator of the Pet Assisted Therapy program at the Peninsula Humane Society & SPCA. She has a PhD in education, counseling psychology from Stanford University and is a licensed psychologist in private practice. Marivic specializes in treating children and adolescents with anxiety/panic, phobias, and grief/loss, and is an accredited provider for the Triple P Positive Parenting Program.

———————

When asked, "What do you want to be when you grow up?" my response was always "A veterinarian." If you liked animals, this was the go-to career choice. Fast forward to today, I coordinate the Pet Assisted Therapy (PAT) program at the Peninsula Humane Society & SPCA (PHS/SPCA) and am a licensed psychologist in private practice. My career in human animal interaction (HAI) can be explained by the Happenstance Learning Theory, where "the career destiny of each individual cannot be predicted in advance, but is a function of countless planned and unplanned learning experiences beginning at birth" (Krumboltz, 2009). My dissertation adviser developed this theory, and it reflects my career journey and will likely reflect yours.

My experience with the human-animal bond began in childhood. Growing up shy, the animals in my life were a source of comfort—from Speedy, the rabbit, to Bubba, the Irish setter. My positive relationships with animals led me to volunteer with dogs and injured wildlife and complete a veterinary externship in high school. All signs seemed to point to a career in veterinary medicine. However, the truth was that I did not enjoy the natural sciences nor was I particularly good at them. I felt lost and defeated. Then, a chance encounter happened. During my first year at Wellesley, I heard one of my floormates talking excitedly about a psychology class. This moment led me to take that class, major in psychology, and pursue graduate degrees at Harvard and Stanford. While deciding what to research for my dissertation, another opportune moment happened. A classmate handed me his copy of *Between Pets and People: The Importance of Animal Companionship* (Beck & Katcher, 1996) which describes how animals impact people's emotional and physical health. I realized I could combine my passion for helping children and adolescents exposed to trauma and my love for animals. My dissertation examined how an animal-assisted intervention (AAI) involving a therapy rabbit team could support youth exposed to community violence.

Opportunities arose within the realm of HAI—including the ability to co-author a chapter on the human–animal bond, attend conferences, be an ad hoc reviewer for the HAI bulletin, and create a blog. When I began my private practice, my dog Bay, a rat terrier, assisted me with clients with dog phobias. During this time, I missed volunteering with animals and began working with injured and orphaned wildlife at PHS/SPCA. I then learned of an internship there involving the PAT program. This internship led to my current staff position as a PAT coordinator, a job that I love. I directly over-see the program and manage the volunteer handler-animal teams who pro-vide animal-assisted activities (AAA) and animal-assisted therapy (AAT) in the community. The teams bring comfort and stress relief to children, adults, and seniors in a variety of facilities including schools, libraries, assisted liv-ing, hospice, behavioral health, hospitals, and county jails. I recruit handler-animal teams after they have passed the American Kennel Club's (AKC) Canine Good Citizen (CGC) test, screen handlers through phone inter-views, and conduct animal temperament evaluations with behaviorists.

I also conduct handler trainings to address the safety, health, and welfare of the therapy animals, schedule shadowing and mentoring sessions, and maintain documentation for team certification. My work extends beyond the office as I conduct site visits in the community and establish relationships with new facilities. The most rewarding aspect of my job is seeing the PAT teams in action, from making patients smile to relieving student stress before final exams. I also enjoy training handlers and watching the handler-animal teams grow and become more confident as partners. Working for a non-profit, however, can be financially challenging. While PHS/SPCA provides good compensation and benefits, the San Francisco bay area is one of the most expensive places in the US in which to live. I am fortunate to be able to supplement my PHS/SPCA income with my work as a psychologist in private practice.

Part of my job involves speaking engagements, something I have found surprisingly rewarding. Whether talking with older adults about their con-nections with animals, mental health professionals interested in the benefits of the human–animal bond, or students and faculty at a university in the Philippines seeking to integrate AAIs into their counseling program, I am reminded of HAI's universality. If you are interested in pursuing a career in HAI, I would recommend you shadow a handler-animal team on a visit, observe a temperament evaluation, or interview a program coordinator from a therapy animal program. Volunteering for an animal welfare organi-zation is a great way to learn about volunteer services and gain knowledge about canine body language and stress signals, both of which are critical to know when working with dogs in AAIs. Finally, I would recommend enrolling in a professional development certificate or graduate program.

I learned about the ethics involved with AAIs and prioritizing therapy animals' safety, health, and welfare through a certificate program at the Institute for Human-Animal Connection at the University of Denver.

My story is an example of how a career path is not a straight line but instead curved with many windy roads. There is not a specific route you need to pursue. Follow your instincts and intuition. I did an unpaid internship in volunteer services which led to my current position. Like our animal partners, we cannot predict where things will go, but by listening, being curious, open and flexible, the next opportunity in HAI is just around the corner.

References

Beck, A. M., & Katcher, A. H. (1996). *Between pets and people: The importance of animal companionship.* West Layfayette, IN: Purdue University Press.

Krumboltz, J. D. (2009). The happenstance learning theory. *Journal of Career Assessment,* *17*(2), 135–154. https://doi.org/10.1177/1069072708328861

37 A Look Into Animal Assisted Interventions Abroad

Entrecanes Association in Northern Spain

Carolina Duarte-Gan

Carolina Duarte-Gan is a certified clinical psychologist and PhD candidate who is researching human animal interactions in children with autism and their families. She provides clinical services with her dogs in Northern Spain. Additionally, she is a co-founder and member of the board of Association Entrecanes, an organization that focuses on Animal Assisted Interventions (AAI).

Welcome to Asturias—Northern Spain, a unique region filled with rainy days, mountains, green fields, and one million people living in three major cities as well as an infinity of small villages; probably not what you imagine when you hear about Spain. It is here where I helped establish Entrecanes Association, a non-profit organization working on AAI, created in 2012.

Entrecanes Association began as a way to involve, in both traditional and less structured settings, human animal interactions in mental health and education. Our goals include improving our clients' quality of life, through human-dog interactions, by helping them achieve their therapeutic, educational or personal goals. We also conduct research pertaining to establishing best practices and guidelines for AAI. Our teams are multidisciplinary, including mental health, educational and social workers as well as veterinarians, dog trainers and administrative personnel. Every staff member has a degree that allows them to work in the fields aforementioned as well as training in AAI and/or anthrozoology. Since the beginning, welfare of our canine working companions has been a priority; therefore, we base our methodology on a square model for our sessions that ensures equal attention and consideration for each of the four critical components: client, dog, human professional and handler.

Our sessions are held in different settings: the Entrecanes Association center, schools, private businesses and homes. My day starts by getting the dogs ready and reviewing the scheduled sessions with the dog handler. Driving to a session can take between 20–60 minutes, so is important to help my canine partner relax, something I do with scent work. Typical interventions with clients range from individual sessions of 20 minutes to hour-long group sessions. After each session, I spend time helping the dog de-stress and evaluate the session. Then, that dog can rest and I prepare for next session with a different dog. In addition to this field work, I spend time completing case reviews, attending professional AAI conferences and presentations, or teaching AAI related courses to other professionals. Every day is a learning experience in the field of AAI.

Nonetheless, there are several challenges to offering AAI in Spain: the lack of a unified field and common definitions (including what is and what is not AAI), available certification and educational opportunities, and general public awareness. The fact that AAI is viewed as a complementary service makes it expendable when funds are scarce. But do not let this discourage you. Efforts are being made to improve research funding and public education around AAI.

Despite these challenges, there are many rewarding parts of my job: the clients, the dogs and the bond they create. That is why I work with Entrecanes: to see elderly people work with the dogs to maintain their cognitive functions improving their quality of life; kindergarten children develop empathy; grade school children learn how to better communicate; at risk youth learn how to cope with being bullied; or survivors of breast cancer or gender violence cope with their current stressors. These interactions, for me, make it all worth it. It is this witnessing of the bond made between these dogs and clients that inspires me to continue working in this field, always pushing to do better and reach additional potential clients in need.

Suggested Skills and Education

From an education standpoint, you need to have a degree that allows you to work in health, education or a social setting. Many people are drawn to AAI work, but do not have adequate training. Second, I suggest that anthrozoology and ethology courses are a must. They give you the scientific background knowledge of human animal interaction and animal behavior needed for this type of work. University courses are a great (and safe) way to start. There is an abundance of information about these types of courses offered by international organizations such as International Association of Human-Animal Interaction Organizations (IAHAIO), The International Society for Anthrozoology (ISAZ) and the International Society for Animal Assisted Therapy (ISAAT).

It is also advisable to contact a local AAI organization and ask if they have any practical training or volunteering opportunities available. This type of experience will give you an insight on the day-to-day routine and if this type of work is a good fit for you. It is helpful to gain as broad of experience as possible; working with different animals, facilities, organizations and professionals can help you better evaluate how you want to incorporate AAI into your work. Other competencies needed for this type of work include teamwork and effective communication skills. You must also be adept at adapting to different situations and unforeseen events. If after getting a variety of experiences, AAI still seems like a good fit, I suggest you reach for what you want—and get ready for the journey of your life.

38 Program Design, Implementation, and Management

Human-Animal Interactions

Carrie Nydick Finch

Carrie Nydick Finch MS, LCSW, is a licensed clinical social worker and is certified in Animal-Assisted Activities, Therapy, and Learning from the University of Denver as well as a therapeutic horseback riding instructor with PATH International. Carrie is the Program Director at PAWS NY, a nonprofit organization that helps mobility-impaired, low-income individuals keep their pets at home. She is also an adjunct faculty member at Columbia University School of Social Work.

My entire life, I have been drawn to animals. Besides becoming a veterinarian, I presumed that spending time with them would always be a hobby. It took years for me to realize otherwise.

Immediately after graduating college, I was offered an opportunity to live and work in Panama, and not yet being certain of my career objectives, I accepted. Living in Panama forced me to examine my core values, and I realized I needed to pursue a career that contributed to the advancement of social justice. That became my guiding principle and when I returned home, I began the journey toward becoming a social worker.

For several years, I gained experience in the social service field before joining the Master's in social work program at Columbia University. In school, I chose the track that focused on advanced generalist practice and programming, developing skills like needs assessments and program planning and design, as well as development and grant writing on top of the clinical foundations of social work.

Throughout the years of my early career, I gained invaluable clinical skills and insight, but always felt personally unfulfilled. I started investigating the field of Human-Animal Interactions, and the research up to that point, although limited in scope, was generating fascinating results. This exploration reinforced what I already knew anecdotally: the bond between humans and animals can be incredibly powerful. I recognized that this field could be the perfect amalgamation of my interests and my skills. I went on to complete a certificate program in Animal Assisted Activities, Teaching and Learning at the University of Denver, and started looking for jobs.

Soon after, I learned about PAWS NY, whose mission is to keep people and companion animals together by providing free pet care services to individuals who are unable to do it themselves. Volunteers visit clients dealing with mobility impairments due to advanced age, illness, or injury, and provide pet care. PAWS NY was searching for someone to join the Founder/ Executive Director, who had just transitioned to full-time. The organization was specifically looking to bring on a social worker, who would have the skills and training necessary to manage services for a complex demographic of clients. In addition to being familiar with the research that confirms various emotional and physical benefits pets can provide for people struggling with many of the issues PAWS NY clients face, I immediately felt personally and powerfully connected to the mission. It seemed like kismet that PAWS NY was looking for a social worker, and that I was able to bring a unique set of skills around program design and implementation to the table.

As Program Director for PAWS NY, every day is different as I oversee a variety of programs including a very large volunteer pet care program, veterinary care and pet pantry programs, and an emergency foster care program. I am responsible for relationships with programmatic partners, and ensuring that our clients receive high-quality, effective services. As a social worker, I am also able to assist programmatic staff by providing clinical guidance, including client behavioral concerns, client and volunteer dynamics, and crisis intervention. Due to our size, with just five full-time staff, we can be responsive and agile. I can see a programmatic need and address it quickly. In the seven years since I joined PAWS NY, the organization's budget has grown over 400%, allowing us to continually expand and refine service provision and offer new programs. For example, after identifying an immense need, I was able to develop and implement the only program in New York City solely focused on providing emergency foster care for pets whose guardians are unexpectedly hospitalized. We partner with hospital staff and social service providers, assessing pets for placement and recruiting and rapidly coordinating volunteer foster homes.

Working for a small nonprofit means that you can hear directly from clients who, without your program, may have been separated from their sole companion and source of support. It is remarkable to know that you personally contributed to keeping their family together, keeping a pet out of the overburdened shelter system, and enhancing the client's emotional well-being.

Conversely, when you have such a high level of ownership, a failure can feel not only professionally painful but also personally devastating. If you are passionate about this work, you will likely take on too much both materially and emotionally. As any social service professional, you are more susceptible to burnout or compassion fatigue due to the high level of empathy required by your job. A small organization won't necessarily have the infrastructure, like clinical supervision and expert guidance, to support you. You must make use of your professional skills to seek out self-care resources.

There are countless paths to a career in the field of Human–Animal Interactions. I have found that the path is rarely linear, but you will learn something about yourself and/or the work at every turn. Numerous experiences and positions can coalesce to deliver a rewarding career. I have found fulfillment and balance as a licensed clinical social worker and Program Director at PAWS NY, while also teaching at Columbia University School of Social Work, and being a therapeutic horseback riding instructor. For me, this variety keeps the work interesting, gratifying, and meaningful.

39 Experiences in Animal-Assisted Interventions (AAI)

Practice, Research, and Teaching

Patricia Flaherty Fischette

Patricia Flaherty Fischette, PhD, is an Animal-Assisted Interventions (AAI) researcher and clinical social worker. She works as a clinician supporting young adults with intellectual disabilities and is the Research Fellow for SoulPaws Recovery Project, the only outpatient AAI for individuals struggling with food and body image issues. She is teaching the first-ever class on AAI at the Bryn Mawr College Graduate School of Social Work and Social Research exploring AAI and trauma.

My interest in AAI developed from my experience growing up in a family that always included animals—dogs, rabbits, hamsters, snakes, bearded dragons, and turtles. As I pursued my social work career, the interplay of animals and healing surfaced in many ways. Specifically, in my clinical work with individuals struggling with eating disorders, a client with an eating disorder said the only thing keeping her alive was her dog. Given the theoretical postulations about eating disorders manifesting as an all-consuming relationship (Schaefer, 2009), it led to thoughts about the relational expectations of humans versus animals. Can an animal prompt less relational expectations thereby accessing emotions and affect in a less threatening way but, at the same time, offer the relational unconditionality desired by individuals struggling with eating disorders? This began the conceptual foundation upon which I built my research of AAI and eating disorders.

My research was the first study that investigated the connection between attachment, affect regulation, eating disorders, and AAT. Forty in-depth semi-structured interviews were conducted with self-identified female adults who were diagnosed with an eating disorder in the last ten years and who used AAT in their eating disorder treatment (75% Canine-Assisted Therapy; 25% Canine and Equine-Assisted Therapy). Eating disorders can be conceptualized as a cluster of vulnerabilities related to affect, attachment, and difficulties in self-regulatory functions (Petrucelli, 2014). Exploration of AAI with eating disorders is an innovative concept connecting their commonality, as both AAI and eating disorders have an impact on affect regulation.

My Background

I received my PhD in social work from Bryn Mawr College Graduate School of Social Work and Social Research, and I am a licensed clinical social worker (LCSW). Currently, I am an adjunct professor at Bryn Mawr College Graduate School of Social Work and Social Research and teaching the first-ever class on AAI. The class, AAI and Trauma, is an elective for graduate-level social work students. Additionally, I am the Research-Scholar for SoulPaws Recovery Project, Inc. and facilitator for SoulPaws Animal-Assisted Activity Workshops for individuals struggling with food/body image issues.

My day-to-day work is extremely varied but always includes thoughts about human-animal interactions. My work generally falls into three domains: researcher on AAI and eating disorders; facilitator of AAI for individuals with eating disorders/food and body issues; and teacher about AAI. In my researcher role, I spend time working on conference presentations to disseminate information about AAI and eating disorders. In addition, I work on publishing my research findings in academic journals. In my facilitator of AAI and eating disorders role, I am spearheading the first SoulPaws Animal-Assisted Activity Workshops in Philadelphia. In doing so, I have been partnering with AAI organizations, reviewing and updating the Soul-Paws workshop curriculum, and facilitating the workshops. In my teacher role, I teach a class on AAI and trauma. This is the first time Bryn Mawr is offering a class on AAI, so the purpose of the class has been an exploration of AAI (theory and practice). In my role as teacher, I design the course, coordinate speakers for the class, and craft assignments that help students wrestle with current AAI issues (ex: evaluate an AAI intervention).

Rewarding and Challenging Parts of My Job

It has been extremely rewarding to learn about the ways in which AAI has positively impacted individuals (specifically, individuals who struggled with eating disorders) when other forms of treatments/treatment providers had been ineffective. Through my research and supported by theories of attachment/affect regulation, AAI may provide opportunities for individuals with eating disorders to experience healing. One participant in my research said about AAT, "it's almost like Neosporin on the wound. It's just like healing it."

The biggest challenge with my job has been the ability to secure research funding for qualitative research in AAI. AAI research requires resilience, determination, and perseverance. Therefore, funding for research may take time, and the need for flexibility (ex: collaborations with other colleagues you did not anticipate) and willingness to promote your research in different ways (ex: sharing my research in a book about HAI careers) are steps in the right direction.

Current Projects and Future Goals

I am working with the Bryn Mawr Graduate School of Social Work and Social Research to offer another class on AAI and expand the current syllabus. In addition, I am looking into offering more SoulPaws workshops and partnering with college counseling centers and/or health centers to offer other animal-assisted activities. My long-term goal is to open a treatment center for individuals with eating disorders where animal-assisted therapy is an integral part of the treatment process and/or develop an AAI program that can be used in eating disorder treatments.

References

Petrucelli, J. (Ed.). (2014). *Body-states: Interpersonal and relational perspectives of the treatment of eating disorders*. New York: Routledge and Taylor & Francis Group.

Schaefer, J. (2009). *Goodbye ed, hello me: Recover from your eating disorder and fall in love with life*. New York: McGraw-Hill.

40 Human-Animal Interaction on the New York City Subway (Long Before Pizza Rat)

Maya Gupta

Maya Gupta, PhD, is the Senior Director of Research for the American Society for the Prevention of Cruelty to Animals, where she leads a team focused on research and program evaluation efforts in the areas of cruelty/disaster response, public policy, community engagement, animal behavior, and equine and farm animal welfare. She is also an adjunct faculty member for the University of Florida Veterinary Forensic Sciences Program and the master's program in anthrozoology at Canisius College, and a guest lecturer/supervisor for the Veterinary Social Work Program at the University of Tennessee.

My career in the field of HAI began one June afternoon inside a hot, sweaty #1 train below Broadway, as my eyes lit on an ad for a domestic violence crisis hotline: "Has your partner ever threatened or hurt your pet?" As a recent college graduate who planned to apply to Ph.D. programs in clinical psychology but hadn't yet identified her intended area of focus (an existential crisis one must resolve before writing a successful application), I was lucky to have my lightbulb moment there in that train. I loved animals, and even fostered cats in my miniscule Manhattan apartment—but never realized I could fuse that extracurricular passion with my professional path. I wish this book had been around back then!

Before I committed to devoting the next however-many years of my life to studying the connection between animal cruelty and domestic violence, I wanted to be sure that my efforts would have potential value for both human service and animal protection agencies. A few phone calls led me to Dr. Stephanie LaFarge, a psychologist at the American Society for the Prevention of Cruelty to Animals, who confirmed that the issue needed more attention from researchers and the field as a whole.

Focus on research that could be applied "in the trenches" guided me through my master's and doctoral work at the University of Georgia. I craved a home in the nonprofit sector, where I could design real-life solutions to problems illuminated by my studies. I became a volunteer, Board member, Board President, and ultimately the first Executive Director of Ahimsa

House, an organization that helps human and animal victims of domestic violence across Georgia reach safety together.

It often felt lonely during graduate school as the only person doing "animal stuff," and at Ahimsa House as the only program of its kind in the state. Yet, when I looked further afield, I found more and more psychologists, psychology students, and others who were interested in human–animal interaction (HAI). Pursuing these connections gave me a support network and introduced me to fellow psychologists who would be instrumental in my career path. These included Dr. Mary Lou Randour, then at Humane Society of the United States and now at the Animal Welfare Institute, who enlisted me in her quest to form a section on HAI in the American Psychological Association. We made the dream a reality in 2008: the field now has a dedicated forum within APA.

My next stop was the Animals & Society Institute: founded by a psychologist, and right up my alley in having developed the first intervention programs for animal cruelty. As Executive Director, I had the opportunity to explore a broader range of HAI topics, and to get back to my scientific roots through producing two academic journals and a variety of student-focused programs. As I had at Ahimsa House, I also launched an internship program to draw more students into HAI and offer them exposure to the nonprofit sector.

In the last few years, my path has brought me back to where it all began: I currently serve as Senior Director of Research for the ASPCA, where I had that first chat with a psychologist over 20 years ago. As part of a 14-person Strategy & Research team, my projects cover everything from veterinary forensics to animal behavior to equine welfare. Our task is to use data to guide organizational direction and decision-making, as well as to drive change and action in animal welfare. My experience designing and evaluating nonprofit service programs comes in just as handy as my formal research training, since we produce both internally focused program evaluations and externally focused research. Even as a big organization, we can't do it all—so, like any nonprofit, we must constantly prioritize our work and remain vigilant against mission drift. But doing so helps ensure that we're producing the most impactful research we can with the resources we have, which brings me to the most rewarding part of my job: targeting our work toward systemic change that can make a difference on a big scale.

If you're considering a future where you can make a difference in HAI, perhaps specifically in the nonprofit sector, here's my advice:

1. Please do! Some truly exciting work is happening at nonprofits, and your skills—whether inclined toward clinical work, research, or both—can be a great contribution.
2. Embrace the non-linear path—or forge paths of your own. Your dream job at your favorite nonprofit doesn't exist yet? Getting involved in a different role, as a means of building your familiarity with (and to)

the organization, may pay dividends down the road—and, meanwhile, you're still contributing to the same mission. If circumstances allow, you might also see if you can start by volunteering or externing there (even if the organization has no formal program of this type). You may be able to turn it into official employment down the road, even if you wind up writing the job description for your own position (as I did at Ahimsa House).

3. Similarly, don't be daunted if you don't have a degree in nonprofit administration, law, fundraising, marketing, or any of the other fields that might seem like prerequisites. There's much to be said for learning via osmosis and resources like The Foundation Center and BoardSource.

4. Don't go it alone. There are great networks and resources to support you. And I'm always delighted to hear from colleagues at any stage in their careers, so please reach out if I can ever be helpful to you in your journey!

41 A Fair Shake for Youth

Helping Middle School Kids Connect With Dogs—While Discovering Their Own Best Selves

Audrey Hendler

Audrey Hendler is the Founder and Executive Director of Fair Shake for Youth, a nonprofit organization that brings hands-on therapy dog programs to underserved middle school students in New York City. She is also a Certified Professional Dog Trainer (CPDT), Pet Partner therapy dog evaluator, and AKC CGC evaluator.

Until I was 38, the only pets I owned were two turtles, JFK and Acrobat. I'd wanted a dog when I was a kid, but my brother was allergic. When I was studying economics at Cornell, I would always stop and pet Reds, a golden retriever who would lie outside the library while his owner was inside studying, but he wasn't mine. After I earned my MBA at the University of Michigan and began working as a marketer in the financial services industry, I didn't think I had the time. Finally, I adopted a yellow Lab, Gator, from a neighbor who was moving to Australia. Having a dog was even better than I'd imagined.

Shortly thereafter, I began volunteering with Puppies Behind Bars, a program in which prison inmates raise service and explosive detection dogs. By then I was running my own marketing consultancy, so my schedule was flexible. Whenever they asked if I could help, I said yes, including when they asked me if I wanted to teach the inmates how to train the puppies in their care. I hadn't taught before, and I wasn't a dog expert; I learned on the job. As it turned out, the puppies did most of the work for me, as they showed the prisoners that they were capable and compassionate people who could learn and grow, be resilient, and give back. My experience with this program led me to create the program A Fair Shake for Youth, in which trained instructors and volunteer therapy dog teams work with kids in middle schools in underserved New York City communities to help them build the social and emotional skills they need to be successful both in an out of school. Interacting with the dogs over the course of the ten-week curriculum shows the kids that they are both loving and lovable—and helps them build the skills they will need to navigate life's challenges.

To prepare, I spent a year attending conferences, participating in dog training workshops; taking courses at John Jay College of Criminal Justice; and networking with professionals in the criminal justice system, the American Society for the Prevention of Cruelty to Animals, and Green Chimneys, a school that focuses on animal-assisted activities for children with special needs. Fair Shake's first program worked with teens involved in the juvenile justice system, but we quickly saw that the opportunity was much broader. For 18 months we tested programs in elementary, middle, and high schools before concluding that we could have the greatest impact on middle school students, who are just beginning the critical transition to adulthood. Children ages 11 to 13 are young enough to want to have a relationship with both dogs and their handlers while also having the cognitive maturity to be able to relate the dogs' experiences to their own.

Early on I recognized that A Fair Shake would have to be my full-time job for it to succeed. Though I was prepared to not draw any salary for the first several years, I didn't realize how challenging starting an organization from scratch would be. My business experience was instrumental in its eventual success; I knew how to meet deadlines, manage projects and budgets, and work with a wide range of stakeholders. I also sought help in critical areas where I did not have experience—grant-writing, fundraising, and working with a board of directors. Ultimately, I found the courage to proceed because people believed in the mission and in me. At first, my focus was on program development and logistics—how do we get volunteers, build school partnerships, get the dogs to school, and develop a curriculum? Now my focus is more on building strategies and ensuring long-term sustainability.

I attribute much of our success to the confluence of two factors: the increasing demand for social and emotional learning, and the recognition and acceptance of the help that dogs can provide. It is critical, however, that we recognize and respect the fact that the vast majority of dogs are *not* well-suited to this work—and that we consider the emotional and physical needs of the few who are.

I am thankful that I can use the skills I learned in the for-profit world to work with so many people who care about kids and appreciate the power that dogs have to make a difference in their lives. I leave you with the story of Roberto. During the last week of his program, Roberto walked up to Brenda and her dog Sam and said, "Sam came from a shelter and she turned out okay. Well, I live in a shelter. Do you think I will be okay?"

"You are already more than okay," Brenda responded.

When I began my career, I never would have expected that I would end up finding and following my passion as I have with A Fair Shake. I went the traditional route (something that hardly seems to exist anymore), but I ended up on a very different path. Stories like Roberto's keep me going.

42 Kids and Dogs. Sounds Easy, Right?

Terri, Copper and Shay Hlava

Terri Hlava and her Literate Labrador teammates work with school children, examining how their beliefs about learning change when they work with therapy dogs. Additionally, Terri co-founded the non-profit research organization H.A.B.I.T.A.T. (Human Animal Bond In Teaching And Therapies), researches in under-resourced schools, and teaches Disabilities Studies in the School of Social Transformation at Arizona State University.

I can honestly say that I love my career. My teammates and I have worked in schools for 30 years, examining how children's beliefs about learning change when they work in small groups teaching a therapy dog lessons. Along with our teammates, I co-founded the non-profit research organization H.A.B.I.T.A.T. (Human Animal Bond In Teaching And Therapies). We research in under-resourced schools and teach Disabilities Studies in the School of Social Transformation at Arizona State University.

In this field, there's something to love every day, but there's no such thing as an average day when you work with young children and dogs. Sure, you establish a basic routine with certain rules about interacting nicely together, and yes, you might have a schedule, and even a lesson plan in mind when you begin the day, but, if you do your job well, then no two days are ever the same. And no days are average. Even with behavioral expectations firmly in place, the days necessarily unwind organically because every student brings different gifts and challenges. And your canine teammate will respond accordingly, empowering the shy student to participate, encouraging the student with speech/language differences to communicate effectively, and it all happens as you're trying to cover some specific information or other important aspect of instruction that you'd so carefully planned. It doesn't even matter what learning label is displayed on the classroom door, e.g. autism spectrum, learning dis/abilities, English language learners, etc. Just remember that if there are kids and dogs, it's going to be wonderful and surprising, and in some ways unplannable, so flexibility is crucial. It allows you to recognize the true potential of these honest authentic learning opportunities.

Suggestions on an Experiential Exercise

So, can you juggle? Balancing flexibility with preparation initially may seem like a juggling act. It takes courage, commitment, and practice to build this skill, so we recommend interviewing, observing, and volunteering with working dog teams to get a better feel for the job before you and your canine companion enter a classroom together so that you can make the most of every minute, planned or spontaneous. Establish strong, trusting relationships with your colleagues and administrator(s). Learn everything you can. Read the research. Check out Division 17 of the American Psychological Association (www.div17.org/sections/human-animal-interaction/) and HABRI (Human Animal Bond Research Initiative habricentral.org). Visit, or virtually visit, working models of human–animal interaction including Green Chimneys, with two campuses in New York (greenchimneys. org), and Kids and Canines in Tampa, Florida (kidsandcanines.org). Take a course. More and more colleges and universities are offering continuing education, certifications, minors and degrees in this field. Consider joining a reputable therapy dog organization that provides insurance for your visits. And, speaking of those visits, the requisite preparation varies. Some therapy dog programs require at least one year of experience before even submitting an application. Other programs only require a copy of the dog's current vaccine record and no additional experience, training or documentation. Sometimes, you'll be the ones designing the program. So, the answer is yes. You can juggle. With some preparation and practice. The average dog can juggle too (at least when it comes to accommodating the schedules of a personal human)

What else do we know about average dogs? Correct! No such beings exist. Dogs, like children, are unique. But there are some strategies that working teams use to begin stacking up those early successes. For instance, if you're the human in the equation, and you are partnered with a therapy dog, then make sure that this dog is happy and healthy and loves working. Like you and your students, dogs love learning too, but when your partner needs a day off, consider a classroom activity that incorporates social and cognitive skills. Encourage the students to make cards for their absent friend, conveying the idea that we all need personal time and space and a measure of autonomy in our lives.

Special Words of Warning or Encouragement

Finally, just as you protect your partner's well-being, you may need to protect your heart too. For example, as the human on the team, you might glean disturbing information as a child confides in the classroom canine. You may be required to report the information to authorities. So, be aware and open, lest you learn something that could change a child's world. Every encounter could change your world too, so take the time to take good care of each other.

We wish you purpose, perseverance, and all the best as you embrace the field of human-animal interaction, well-equipped to make a lasting, positive difference. Begin. Change the world . . . Share your strategies, successes and setbacks. Learn. Practice. Teach. Refine. Repeat.

43 Working With a Facility Dog in a Veterans Affairs Hospital

Elizabeth Holman

Elizabeth Holman, PsyD, is the palliative care psychologist at the Rocky Mountain Regional VA Medical Center and an assistant adjunct professor in the Department of Medicine, University of Colorado School of Medicine. Elizabeth is joined in her work by Tootsie, a facility dog who brings comfort and support to the veterans they serve.

———————

When I tell people about my job, they murmur sympathetically, "That sounds so hard." I work with veterans who are seriously ill and at end of life, but in truth, I love it. Being a palliative care psychologist at the Veterans Affairs hospital is everything I've ever hoped for in a career—challenging, fascinating, and deeply meaningful. There are definitely tears. But the work is also filled with laughter, growth, and flashes of grace. Best of all, it also involves dog fur.

My path was anything but linear. With degrees in religion and theology, I've always been interested in what matters most to people. I worked in education policy, then did mediation and child advocacy in high-conflict divorce. I entered a PsyD program in my late 30s, hoping to find a career that fed both my spirit and practical needs. Health psychology classes and a geropsychology practicum rekindled my interest in the workings of body and brain. After an internship at a Veterans Affairs hospital (VA) and post-doctorate position on a bone marrow transplant unit, I was fortunate to return to the VA as the psychologist on the fledgling palliative care team.

I had joyful companions on this path—service dog puppies. My spouse and I raised five puppies for Canine Companions for Independence (CCI). Volunteer raisers have pups from 8 weeks to 18 months, teaching basic commands and socialization skills. I took these pups to stores and movies, courthouses, difficult interviews, and psychology classes. I saw that in stressful settings people soon were smiling and connecting. One of our puppies became a facility dog, trained like a service dog but partnered with an able-bodied handler in their work. I dreamed of one day having my own facility dog.

First, though, I had to focus on my new job. I had never done palliative care, and the team had never had a psychologist. The VA has all the drawbacks of working for a vast bureaucracy and some of my most teeth-grinding moments have come from these structural challenges. But it also has a nationwide community that helped our interdisciplinary team develop my role.

My days include assessing patients and families' mood and coping; facilitating family meetings; assessing decision-making capacity; supporting patients and families; and helping the team understand the psychological factors affecting our patients. I work primarily on inpatient medical wards, but also see outpatients for individual therapy.

As I became more comfortable in my role, my thoughts returned to the potential benefits of a facility dog partner. Veterans seen in palliative care are often in pain, frightened, and suspicious of the VA generally and psychology in particular. My experience told me that our veterans would connect with a dog. However, there were no facility dogs in acute medical settings in any other VA. I proposed my idea, and although it was well received by leadership, it still took a year to satisfy safety and cleanliness concerns before I could even apply.

After a lengthy application process and two weeks of Team Training at Canine Companions I was matched with Waffle, a yellow Lab-golden cross. Through the years of my partnership with facility dogs I have continued to learn from classes in animal-assisted therapy, reading, and consulting with other facility dog handlers. Waffle and her successor, Tootsie, make literally every day better for me, my team, our patients, and colleagues. These dogs open doors for our team as veterans who are unsure about us allow the dog in, giving us an opportunity to join with them and offer care. They provide a moment of softness, sweetness, and heart connection that heals patients and staff alike.

In my current position, I rarely work evenings or weekends. But the job involves bearing witness to grief, loneliness, and suffering, plus tremendously meaningful moments. This affects not just my work, but how I move through the world. Learning how and when to metabolize these emotions with colleagues, family, and a therapist is an ongoing challenge. I also have a responsibility to my canine partner, including monitoring her well-being and ensuring she gets exercise and play, both of which take me out of myself and remind me to give myself the same care.

This career choice can demand all your brain and all your heart. It also requires patience; it can be a long time between the idea and reality of an animal partner. Plenty of people, rules, and structures will say it won't work. During my long process of trying to get approval for a facility dog, a friend said, "It seems you're in the grip of something larger than yourself." I did feel there were forces beyond me moving to bring a facility dog to our VA. That kept me asking and working until we outlasted the naysayers. If you sense that your path includes working in human-animal interaction, keep stepping forward until the road unfolds.

44 An Industry Veterinarian's Perspective on a Career in Human–Animal Interaction

Karyl Hurley

Karyl J. Hurley, DVM, DACVIM, DECVIM-CA, is the Director of Global Scientific Policy and Engagement at Mars, Incorporated. She is currently part of the Mars Global Corporate Scientific and Regulatory Affairs team based in the US. In this role, Karyl provides strategic leadership in the governance of Mars scientific research with human and animal participants. Karyl also manages the Mars Research Review Board which is accountable for ensuring all of our research adheres to robust ethical and scientific standards.

I have had a unique and wonderful journey in the practice and study of human-animal interactions (HAI), and I welcome the opportunity to share my story in hopes that others may be encouraged and know that there is no one right path in finding what you love to do. Following formative years in academia, I have worked over two decades for an industry that at its core feeds people, cares for pets, and seeks to have a positive societal impact.

I am first and foremost a veterinarian, and the health and welfare of pets has been the focus of my career for over three decades. In the years I worked in academia, I loved the work—seeing patients, teaching students, and leading rounds and journal clubs—but the downside was that my patients who, by the nature of referral to a specialist, were very ill, had highly caring owners, but eventually succumbed to their diseases. While helping animals and their families is an awesome reward of being a practicing veterinarian, it is also a common cause of compassion fatigue. When I was offered a role in Scientific Communications for WALTHAM Petcare Science Institute, a division of Mars Incorporated (UK), I learned that I could help pets in other ways. I lectured internationally, and edited and published journals and newsletters focused on pet health. Industry roles can be dynamic and after a few years, I returned to the US to join our Mars Corporate Scientific and Regulatory Affairs team where I help the Mars business understand and address pet health challenges and food safety issues. A highlight of my career in HAI was when we approached the prestigious

Eunice Kennedy Shriver National Institute of Child Health and Human Development (NICHD), found that we shared a common enthusiasm, and entered a public-private-partnership (PPP) to gain momentum for the field. Together, over the past 12 years, we have provided support for workshops and scientific conferences, published three textbooks and numerous journal articles, and provided sustained funding for dozens of research studies. The PPP has encouraged the adaptation of rigorous research designs and methodologies on topics ranging from pet ownership and social isolation to addressing the contributions of service animals to the social functioning of children and military service veterans with post-traumatic stress disorders or PTSD.

Now, as the Mars Global Director of Science Policy and Engagement for the past three years, my role is to ensure the science we do is rigorous, transparent and benefits people, pets and the planet. I engage in many pet health issues and am a point of contact for veterinary and HAI advice and expertise within Mars and for our external partners.

When I reflect on the path to my current position, I find that the role seemed to grow around me rather than having a preconceived vision or trying to master a list of required skills. I do feel, however, that there are some core competencies people who work with animals must have, including compassion, empathy and the ability to communicate well with both people and animals. An industry role in science requires the ability to deal with ambiguity, to assess what is needed and fill the gap, to work well within a team and build an external network of scientific support and knowledge. This role requires filtering and assessing a great deal of information about animals, from scientific publications, news and even social media, and communicating these findings effectively to a global audience. Examples include the public perception of pets—the bond and the benefits of pets for individuals, families and communities. On the rare occasions when there are food safety incidents that affect humans and animals (e.g. zoonoses like salmonella, MRSA or campylobacter, or perceived threats such as COVID-19), I provide technical support and advice on how to best manage people and pet interactions.

My role is global and remotely based from a home office surrounded by my own pets. This is both a wonderful perk and often a challenge as it requires clear separation of personal and professional time and space. I live within reasonable distance to a train station and an airport as travel is necessary to ensure regular meetings with internal teams and scientific colleagues. Compensation is relevant to one's needs, and for me, I was able to pay off my student loans by my early 30s and have all I need to live well and feel comfortable when I retire, hopefully some years from now.

I have been very fortunate in my career and am grateful for the options that were available to me. I have held many varied roles in teaching and industry that have given me great joy in working with animals and their humans. My advice is to have a sense of adventure and do not let fear of the unknown prevent you from taking opportunities as they arise to move, grow, change and redefine how you lead your life. You will learn to know yourself better, what holds your interest and what challenges you. All jobs will change and grow over time, particularly in industry, so learn to find excitement and fulfillment in change.

45 Pick Your Own Adventure, Finding a Career in the Nonprofit World

Emily Patterson-Kane

Emily Patterson-Kane, PhD, is a New Zealander who has gained research and teaching experience in Scotland, Canada, and America. Her core discipline is behavioral psychology with a focus on animal welfare and human-animal interactions. Emily currently works for the American Society for the Prevention of Cruelty to Animals (ASPCA) and has authored articles and chapters on how to provide environmental enrichment, the causes of animal cruelty, and the provision of euthanasia.

My entry point into the field was an undergraduate psychology class presenting a radical behaviorist philosophy of psychology. Despite being desperately unfashionable even then, something about the Skinnerian approach to science really clicked with me. Behaviorist psychology, combined with my interest in animal welfare, mapped out the area where I wanted to have my career.

I earned my graduate degrees focusing exclusively on research (first studying whether chickens can understand TV pictures, and then looking at how to provide and assess environmental enrichment for rats). I then pursued post-doctoral research, studying rat habitat design, assessing the accuracy of human assessments of emotion in pigs, and testing what kinds of enrichment pigs will work hardest for. The role of human-animal interactions crept in along the way.

I remember how, during my PhD, an undergraduate student asked if the rats are happy. It wasn't an uncommon thing for students to ask. We had a stock answer that lab rats were healthy and lived longer than those in the wild and were well cared for. While technically accurate, for a reply by a psychologist in a psychology lab, it was somewhat devoid of . . . psychology. On that one occasion, for some reason, I really heard the question as it was intended—and it occurred to me that I thought the answer was no. Happiness is a little more and different from health, care, and longevity. My career goals changed around that time because I knew I wanted to make things better for animals, make them *happier*. And I wanted more people to take on that goal for the animals in their community and their industries.

My career could have gone a lot of different ways, and the factors that limited my opportunities were as important as the things that inspired me. I started out in research and had a classic academic career in mind, yet I struggled to find a permanent position. I realized it was time to begin looking for work outside of academia. First, I worked as an animal welfare scientist at the American Veterinary Medical Association (AVMA). The month I was offered that job I got two tenure track offers (because apparently the universe is perverse like that) and I turned them down. I second-guessed that decision for many years, but now I am confident it was the right choice for me. Recently I was hired to be a research director at the ASPCA.

I have had many jobs over the last 15 years, and I would have to say that I have really enjoyed my work. It's not that it isn't often frustrating or annoying in some ways, but I believe in the overall goals I am pursuing, I respect the people I work with, and I feel like my work is appreciated and fairly compensated. One of the most important things that I have realized, looking back, is that my discipline identity as a psychologist was very important in giving me the toolkit I needed to do my work. However, out of five previous jobs I have held, only one was advertised as a job for a psychologist. Therefore, I would suggest casting your net wide when searching for vacancies and don't overthink sending in an application if you find something unusual and intriguing.

I would encourage students and early-career people to make sure they keep an open mind about where their career might take them. This might include moving to another country or disciplinary area or looking for opportunities not only in academia but also non-profits, industry, and government or regulatory agencies (and more!). Some of these positions provide a unique opportunity to bring a new perspective and create change—but you must be flexible enough to learn the culture and pick up new skills as you go. (Keep in mind that they use difference terms and definitions in their job ads and may list required qualifications and experience that you don't have, but you can show that you have something equivalent or better or the demonstrated ability to upskill rapidly.) Getting a good education means that you can continue to evolve into new areas; in my case including meta-analysis, project management, qualitative methods, and more! And you can often affect what your jobs duties are once you are in place by showing the relevance of topics that interest you to the organization's strategic goals or mission.

In hindsight I wish I had known more about how to develop a career and realized that it is a skill like any other. I wish I had been more mindful of my options, how to network, and the flexibility of core skills. On the other hand, by doing things the hard way I have developed a real appreciation for having a meaningful job and a comfortable life. My career is a journey now rather than a destination, and I am enjoying the journey.

46 Organized Animal Protection as a Career

Meaning, Mission, and the Academic Contributor

Bernard Unti

Bernard Unti has a PhD in US history. He is the Senior Policy Advisor at the Humane Society of the United States and represents the organization and its affiliates in a range of domestic and global campaigns and initiatives. His interests include the evolution of human attitudes toward animals, the history and sociology of the animal protection movement, the development of petkeeping, animal sheltering and the kindness-to-animals ethic, the humane education of children, and the place of animal protection within American philanthropy.

I often assure individuals seeking work in the field of animal protection that while it might seem like I followed a plan to secure my position with the Humane Society of the United States (HSUS), there was a lot of contingency involved. The HSUS and its affiliates work on a national and global scale to take on some of the most challenging areas of animal cruelty, and I provide enterprise-level communications and policy, strategic, and leadership counsel to its president and CEO. In many respects, I'm a futurist, thinking about how the challenges and opportunities of the animal protection landscape will evolve, and searching across cultures, disciplines, and geographies to identify pathbreaking ideas and solutions to the animal welfare challenges of the coming decades. How remarkable that I do so with a PhD in US history, having followed my passion for studying the humane movement's origins.

But this shouldn't really surprise. One of the best approaches to the present and the future is the past, not only to understand its direct impact but to find analogies that help us to anticipate how current trends or developments may unfold or reshape our circumstances. Only in retrospect can we determine which ideas and approaches have been the most important to our work; at the same time, we cannot know for certain today which contemporary ideas and strategies will prove to be the most valuable in the future.

With that motivation, I write and lecture on the history of animal protection as a social movement, the evolution of humane education, the development of the veterinary profession, and the link between cruelty to animals and interpersonal violence. I speak at professional, academic, and advocacy conferences and events; at colleges and law schools; at humane society functions; and other venues, in the United States and abroad. Finally, I have frequent contact with authors writing on animal protection and have helped to shape some important scholarship and thought. All these things are really satisfying.

I had an innate interest in animals and their welfare as a child, but it was mostly latent until I encountered the animal rights cause in my mid-20s. That did it for me. After a few years spent in grassroots efforts and working at an organization focused on the elimination of animal use in research, testing, and education, my desire to learn more of the movement's history led me to graduate school. It all fell into place. The subject matter compelled my attention, which was the foundation of my success in the dissertation process, and still anchors my long service to the cause of animals.

I spend a lot of time outside of work thinking about issues that require more dedicated problem-solving and engagement. Staying on top of relevant literature is a big part of that. I try to read works of note in a range of academic disciplines, usually on my own time unless I am preparing with intensity for a new talk, webinar, or paper.

I particularly hope to see the integration of more scientists, social scientists, and humanities scholars into humane work. The most typical pathway is for people to cut their teeth on a specific campaign, get a master's degree in animal studies or to go to law school resulting in movement organizations dominated by lawyers, political campaigners, and marketing and development specialists. We need a broader base, and I think that those with backgrounds in the humanities, social science, and the natural sciences will prove to be just as influential and valuable within movement organizations. I say this in part because society is going to need more people qualified to interpret, shape, and manage the increasing incorporation of animals into the social contract and to help us to think about what our responsibilities to animals should and will be like in the future.

To excel in this area of work, writing and communications skills are premium assets, and I advise aspiring professional advocates to take courses or to read good books on writing. I also encourage people to engage directly with organizations, shelters, sanctuaries, and campaigns as a volunteer, donor, or through information interviews or internships (which are of particularly high value). Getting yourself into the workstream of an organization and making yourself visible to key staff members will really pay off.

If you work in a movement organization, you'll find your duties spilling over into your personal time. It's essential to maintain good work-life balance; that's been key to my longevity and tenure. It's necessary to put in extra hours and efforts, but I try to make sure that I do so in moments of true need or in situations that truly have my name on them.

Good self-knowledge and a realistic view of the challenges involved in finding satisfying employment in the field are essential. But few among us will come out wrong in life if we follow our hearts in our choice of work or related pursuits. Anyone with a strong desire to work in animal protection should honor that impulse. It's worth it.

Part IV

Private Practice, AAI Programs

47 Symbiotic Relationship Between Therapist and Co-Therapist

The Story of Emmie

Donna Clarke

Donna Clarke is a licensed clinical professional counselor (LCPC) currently working in private practice. She is a nationally certified counselor (NCC), certi- fied as a clinically trained trauma professional: Level II C-PTSD (CCTP-II) and a certified grief counseling specialist (CGCS) through the International Associ- ation of Trauma Professionals (IATP). Ms. Clarke is a board certified telemental health provider (BC-TMH) through the Center for Credentialing and Educa- tion, Inc. She holds a certificate in Animal Assisted Therapy Training through the University of North Texas Consortium for Animal Assisted Therapy.

The biophilia hypothesis posits an innate connection with earth; a con- nection to nature (Frumpkin, as cited in Fine, 2019). Perhaps that is why many feel a unique inner relationship to water, trees, or wildlife. For me, it has been felt most strongly as a bond with animals. This connection guided me to co-found and operate a non-profit animal hospice for abused and neglected animals. For more than 20 years we travelled with animals toward a life from fear and pain into one of resilience and peace, as they learned to trust again. Some journeyed their lifetimes. Others did not have enough time. All were precious. This experience led me to explore animal assisted activities and interventions while studying to become a licensed clinical professional counselor, design and teach graduate level coursework, and pre- sent at conferences and other institutions, addressing animal assisted thera- pies, activities, and interventions from the perspective of not only potential therapeutic modalities and benefits, but also the welfare of the co-therapist. I have been fortunate to have Emmie, my CTP, to journey with clients in private practice. It is why I feel passionate about sharing in this work.

The bond between therapist and co-therapist represents a truly special and unique relationship, one requiring objective awareness, honest pres- ence, and understanding, as our co-therapist is reliant upon us to provide more than their daily necessities. Emmie brings her present self to the room. It is imperative that I do the same, both as the therapist and as *her* human. Understanding *her* language, in addition to the language of her breed and species, is most important. In that way, her needs are met consistently, con- veniently, and compassionately, whether with a bowl of fresh water, food,

snacks, walks, bathroom breaks, or most importantly, frequent and significant breaks in her day based on her need, not my schedule. Co-therapists
look to us to be able to intuit them on as deep a level as they intuit their
own world, our client and even ourselves. For them, it appears fluid, almost
second nature. For us, it is learned, effortful, and different. With so much of
the language of the living existing in a nonverbal modality, it is very important to be mindful that this is the natural language of the co-therapist. It is a
language we aspire to master.

I have heard it said that non-human animals, specifically dogs, are *Rog-
erian*, existing in the present, providing us with unconditional positive regard.
Put quite simply, they are happy to see us whether we have been gone one
hour or one minute, in dress clothes or sweats, happy or sad. They inform
us of this through visual cues: wagging tails, licks, and friendly barks. They
also provide less subtle cues. This language they use to let us know not only
when they are stressed, but also when they intuit stress in others (Chandler,
2017). These cues provide a wealth of understanding with respect to their
world. They are an invaluable component for not only maintaining awareness of the co-therapist, but also other humans in the room. It can prove
daunting, as we must be present for the client, the co-therapist, and honest
within ourselves to the possibility that it is *we* who are being felt by the co-
therapist, not solely our client.

With respect to non-human animals in session work, through both face-
to-face as well as telemental health, I have the privilege of working alongside my therapy pet, Emmie, a 5.5-pound teacup poodle. Each experience
with Emmie allows clients to glean what they need in the moment, whether
projecting feelings of sadness on Emmie's slower movements, or perceptions
of anxiety through her briskly wagging tail. Connections can be clear and
seemingly immediate for clients who eagerly greet Emmie, asking about her
day, or sharing tools from prior sessions. Connections can be more subtle
for clients who share thoughts of being disconnected from Emmie while
consistently asking about her on days she is not present. My reply: "She
is taking a self-care day. What is your self-care today?" One client shared
thoughts surrounding self-care, and not having the ability to do the same.
What a unique opportunity to explore self-care, mindfulness, and present
focus as well as tools and resources! Some clients enjoy *training* Emmie, and
others share thoughts and feelings otherwise too uncomfortable to discuss
with just another human. Clients appreciate when Emmie sits with them,
fully present, non-judgmental, seeming to innately understand their cir-
cumstance, feelings, and pain. Some enjoy watching her sleep, remarking
on her calmness in the space. Each interaction becomes a unique exten-
sion of the function of the work with Emmie an eager participant in the
learning, sharing, and growth of clients. I am ever mindful that, although
eager to join in the work, *she* has the choice to participate, sit out, or not
attend—always. This component my clients are well aware of and is often
an empowering construct as they themselves often struggle with feelings of
lack of control or empowerment.

Emmie brings such a significant presence to the room; a great deal can be learned from a 5.5-pound dog.

References

Chandler, C. K. (2017). Recognizing stress in therapy animals. In *Animal assisted therapy in counseling* (p. 102). New York: Routledge.

Fine, A. H. (2019). Theories explaining the bond. In A. H. Fine (Ed.), *Handbook on animal assisted therapy: Foundations and guidelines for animal-assisted interventions* (p. 8). Cambridge, MA: Elsevier.

48 A Professional Transformational Journey in the Practice of Animal Assisted Interventions

Molly DePrekel

Molly DePrekel is a psychologist in private practice both at the Midwest Center for Trauma and Emotional Healing and Hold Your Horses. She provides therapy and offers consultation for other professionals in animal assisted interventions (AAI). She holds certifications in sensorimotor psychotherapy, EMDR and yoga. She is also a committee member of the Horses and Humans Research Foundation and faculty at the University of Denver's Institute for Human Animal Connection.

———————

During my undergraduate years, I worked at the Michigan State University horse barns and during the summers, worked at a camp for inner city girls from Detroit. It was my work with these young girls that showed me they had little or no connection with animals and nature. The change in these girls after experiencing animals and nature informed my decision to work at helping people to connect more deeply with themselves through animals and nature. In 1985, while searching the student services books for internships, I found a flyer for a place called Green Chimneys school in New York state. I applied and was accepted as a farm intern. I lived on-site working with residents with severe mental health issues as well as helping with AAI. I have been proud to watch Green Chimneys grow and change into the center it is today.

Post-graduation, I wanted to find a position that included some form of animal assisted therapy. I moved to Minnesota (MN) for work and study at the Center to Study Human-Animal Relationships and the Environment (CENSHARE). My challenge was deciding where I fit in. Was I an occupational therapist, physical therapist, or mental health provider? I chose mental health, completing my graduate work at St. Mary's University, earning a master's in counseling and psychological services.

In my work I hold many roles, all revolving around animal-based therapy work. I have been a therapist in private practice for 29 years in animal assisted therapy and nature-based healing. I was the Clinical Director of a non-profit that specialized in animal assisted therapy and education for professionals. After a ten-year tenure there I established my own practice doing similar work, specializing in trauma healing. Recently I have added consultation services for therapists who want to embark on AAI with their clients.

My therapy dogs are an integral part of my individual therapy with clients in my office setting. For my equine practice, I work with an organization called Hold Your Horses and I provide therapy with the help of horses for adolescents and adults. Within my private practice, I see some clients in my office and others at the barn or in the horse-riding arena. At my private practice office, I include my dogs—whether walking or playing, as well as incorporating other forms of nature-based healing. At the equine barn, I see individual clients and facilitate groups with sexually exploited youth. I currently work with dogs and horses. Currently, I am on the faculty at the University of Denver, School of Social Work, Institute for Human-Animal Interactions and enjoy teaching others.

This work requires an ability to be not only a counselor but animal behaviorist. I highly recommend, especially in sessions that include equines, having other animal handlers to assist. These sentient beings both add to and require more in counseling sessions for which a practitioner must be aware. The animals I work with require a high level of care and responsibility, but the rewards far outstrip the demands. I do not have a traditional 9–5 job. In private practice, I often work later than 5. Due to the population I work with, my groups happen later in the day due to school hours. I may assist on weekends at the barn, conduct workshops for others, or attend trainings around animal interactions. As a college instructor, teaching online, AAI requires weekend and evening work.

I believe there are growth opportunities in the field of AAI as more agencies acknowledge the benefits animals bring. The most important core competencies include mastery as a therapist without the presence of an animal. AAI are an added competency to an established practice of work. It is important to understand and have knowledge of the species with which you will work. This includes knowing animal body language, calming signals and stress responses. This requires more than completing a weekend workshop and should be an area of on-going study for the practitioner. It is important to know how your animal plays and lets off steam. The education to add includes animal behavior, animal handling skills, job shadowing and/or internships that are well established in the work you want to pursue.

I have been challenged and rewarded in my search for mentors. These teachers have now challenged me to train and mentor others. In response to this challenge I started a consultation business with a colleague and fellow instructor at the University of Denver, Alison Leslie LCSW. We offer individual and group consultation in AAI and nature-based healing for others doing this work. Consultation can be done in person, online and in groups.

This work has given me an amazing life journey. I have knocked on many doors, often many times. I tell others to keep searching, screen your teachers and mentors carefully, learn from many people and enjoy learning from animals. Ask questions: discern and critically think about the answers you get. Play along the way, laugh with the animal teachers and when you feel discouraged take a walk in nature, be with the animals and then start again on your journey.

49 A Legal Career With Animals

Akisha Townsend Eaton

Akisha Townsend Eaton is a legislative attorney for Best Friends Animal Society, where she focuses on advancing lifesaving laws and policies, at both the local and state levels, for cats and dogs and the families and community members who care for them. Akisha's international policy experience includes serving as Senior Policy Advisor for World Animal Net, where she advocated for important policy changes in animal welfare in a variety of forums, including at the United Nations.

I became interested in human-animal interaction (HAI) in my senior year of college, after seeing a flyer for an international animal law conference. Having long been passionate about animal welfare, I was intrigued and decided to attend. By the end of the conference, I was set on paving a career in animal law. At that time, however, few full-time legal careers in animal law existed. A few years later, I became one of the first law students to pursue a law degree in hopes of practicing animal law full time. During and after law school, I had an opportunity to pursue two animal welfare fellowships before accepting my first permanent position in the field as a legislative attorney.

One of the most exciting things about my current role as a legislative attorney is that there is no "average day." One day I might be drafting a local or state law to help animals in shelters. The next day, I might be preparing to testify on a bill in the legislature or giving an advocacy presentation to average citizens wishing to get more involved with helping to advance laws to protect animals in their own communities. My current role largely focuses on reducing legal barriers to keeping animals out of shelters. Often, this means amending outdated ordinances that put dogs and cats at high risk of impoundment, and often death, if not able to be returned to an owner in time. One of the most rewarding aspects of my job is knowing that each new law passed has the potential to save thousands of dogs and cats, and offer immediate benefits to the families and community members who care for them. I also get to work alongside amazing community leaders and shelter employees eager to see positive change.

People are often surprised about how much my career intersects with human-animal interactions. However, in my current role, I also enjoy helping people with pets who might find themselves in challenging situations. Efforts to this end might include advocating for new laws to create funding or greater access to low-cost spay/neuter and veterinary care, or for laws and policies to ensure that renters with pets are not unfairly discriminated against in the housing market.

With only a small team with which to interface with the majority of US states and numerous local communities, managing competing deadlines can be challenging, especially when multiple states are in legislative session at the same time of year. My team often needs to focus our efforts on the highest need areas. However, part of our role is to create accessible resources for non-lawyers to be able to effectively engage in the legislative process. We've even had some advocates go on to run for office and win!

My Career Advice

At the time I first began my career, there were only a handful of full-time animal related legal jobs. Since that time, I'm glad to say the landscape has changed dramatically. There are a growing number of students pursuing law school solely to practice animal law, as reflected by a plethora of animal law courses, clinics, fellowships, internships, and full-time opportunities. It is important to remember that there are many subspecialties that fall under the umbrella of animal law that intersect with other areas of law including environmental, consumer protection, and insurance, just to name a few. Similar to every other area of law, it's important to remember that not all animal protection lawyers will find themselves arguing in a courtroom. Though achieving important legal precedents is a critical piece of strengthening the animal law movement, important achievements may also happen through drafting sound contracts and operating standards for and between parties, facilitating important negotiations, and advocating for important policy changes with lawmakers and other officials.

What's more, there are many animal related legal and policy careers for which a law degree may not be required, but may serve as an asset. These include policy specialists and experts, executive director positions, human resource positions, grassroots related positions, and legal support positions. It is important to note that some of these positions offer direct involvement with animal protection issues, while others help support organizations advance their animal protection missions.

For those considering going to law school, I would suggest pursuing a broad-based curriculum, including any animal law courses that may be available, as well as seeking out relevant internships, fellowships, and clerkships. The Animal Legal Defense Fund has a student chapter designed to provide support, advice, and resources to students interested in the field of animal law. They even offer scholarships. For those not immediately going into animal law after graduation, there are countless other ways in which experience in other legal or law-related careers can help prepare a person for an eventual career in animal law. Because law degrees can be expensive and many animal law jobs are at nonprofit organizations, carefully consider programs that offer repayment or forgiveness options for those who pursue public service based careers. Lastly, there are several professional organizations to consider joining, including the American Bar Association's Animal Law Committee, housed within the Tort, Trial, and Insurance Practice Section, as well as the animal law sections of state bar associations. Whichever career path one chooses, a legal career with animals can be a rewarding and life changing experience that makes a lasting impact.

50 Conducting Canine-Assisted Psychotherapy

Betz King

Betz King, PsyD, is a clinical psychologist in Metropolitan Detroit who provides outpatient canine-assisted psychotherapy (CAP). She has a private practice specializing in psycho-spirituality, women's empowerment and existential psychotherapy. Betz has been at the forefront of advocating for and creating emotional support animal guidelines for mental health professionals.

———————

I became interested in CAP after adopting a yellow Labrador named Paisley. Having completed my bachelor and master's degrees in clinical psychology, I was working as a psychotherapist while finishing my doctoral program and didn't want to leave her home every day. My employer let her come to work with me while she was going through Canine Good Citizen and Therapy Dogs International training, and it quickly became evident that Paisley's temperament and intuition made her a valuable addition to psychotherapy sessions. After an early career in community mental health, I moved into private practice, where Paisley and I worked together for almost a decade before she retired. Today, my group psychotherapy practice has four associates and one therapy dog in training, Paisley's great-grandnephew Bodhi.

CAP involves the addition of a canine co-therapist, or therapy dog, into the therapy session (Jones, Rice, & Cotton, 2019). Bodhi and I see between four and eight clients a day and between 15 and 20 clients per week. I bring a psychotherapy client to my office, and Bodhi greets them. If the client chooses to sit on "the dog couch", Bodhi will—if invited—lay next to them. Then the client and I will talk about their therapeutic goals and progress. CAP requires that clients have a goal that Bodhi can assist them with. CAP interventions can be *spontaneous* or animal-led (i.e., Bodhi approaches someone when they're crying), *adjunctive* or facilitator-led (i.e., if a client is highly anxious, I will ask them to match their breathing to Bodhi's as a mindfulness exercise), or *experiential* (participant-led, i.e., the client will invite Bodhi to sit on the couch to take silly selfie photos she can look at when she is feeling sad; Jones et al., 2019). Each intervention is designated to target a specific treatment plan goal.

Most Rewarding Part of Job

There is no greater joy than to see the light bulb go off in a client's head as something inside of them shifts, opening a path to growth and change. CAP is even more heartwarming. While the relationship between therapist and client is one of the most important factors in the healing process (Duncan, 2014), there are elements of the therapy that can only be mutually co-created through the sharing of experiences (Cornelius-White, Kanamori, Murphy, & Tickle, 2018). Adding the here-and-now presence of a dog deepens this mutuality, providing rich opportunities for teachable moments, transferable skills and the magical elixir of all good therapy—unconditional positive regard.

Challenges With Job

While often heartwarming and fun, CAP has challenges as well. The ability to multi-task by tracking and responding to several processes at a time requires greater focus and concentration. For example, if a client is practicing mindfulness by matching his breathing with the dog, the therapist must monitor the client's learning process, the client and dog breathing, the dog's well-being and the treatment goal. In addition to the complexities of the treatment triad, the necessity for frequent breaks and shorter workdays has financial repercussions. There are extra layers of documentation necessary, and clients who are afraid or allergic to dogs will choose to work with someone else. If the canine co-therapist becomes ill or dies, the therapist must process their own feelings of worry and grief while remaining attuned to clients' processes. Almost every facet of CAP is more difficult than traditional psychotherapy.

The field of human animal interaction research, and more specifically animal assisted therapy research, is expanding and this will likely result in future recommendations for canine assisted psychotherapy. While the confidential nature of psychotherapy precludes sitting in on a CAP session, resources such as the *Handbook on Animal-Assisted Therapy: Foundations and Guidelines for Animal-Assisted Interventions* (Fine, 2020), the *Clinician's Guide to Treating Companion Animal Issues: Addressing Human-Animal Interaction* (Blazina & Kogan, 2018) and the Animal Assisted International Standards of Practice (2019) provide substantial guidance for those wishing to enter into the deeply rewarding world of CAP.

References

Blazina, C., & Kogan, L. (Eds.). (2018). *Clinician's guide to treating companion animal issues: Addressing human-animal interaction.* Cambridge, MA: Academic Press.

Cornelius-White, J. H. D., Kanamori, Y., Murphy, D., & Tickle, E. (2018). Mutuality in psychotherapy: A meta-analysis and meta-synthesis. *Journal of Psychotherapy Integration, 28*(4), 489–504. https://doi.org/10.1037/int0000134

Duncan, B. L. (2014). The heart and soul of change. In *On becoming a better therapist: Evidence-based practice one client at a time* (2nd ed., pp. 147–173). American Psychological Association. https://doi.org/10.1037/14392-006

Fine, A. H. (2020). *Handbook on animal-assisted therapy: Foundations and guidelines for animal-assisted interventions*. Cambridge, MA: Academic Press.

Jones, M. G., Rice, S. M., & Cotton, S. M. (2019). Incorporating animal-assisted therapy in mental health treatments for adolescents: A systematic review of canine assisted psychotherapy. *PLoS One, 14*(1), e0210761. https://doi.org/10.1371/journal.pone.0210761

51 Scientist-Practitioner Approach

Harnessing the Power of Equine-Assisted Psychotherapy and Animal-Assisted Interventions in Private Practice

Elizabeth A. Letson

Elizabeth A. Letson, MS, LPCC, is the Founder/Therapist at Eagle Vista Ranch & Wellness Center, where they provide mental health counseling to children, teens, and adults. Here, she incorporates equine-assisted psychotherapy and learning and animal-assisted interventions (EAP/EAL/AAI) into her clinical work with clients. She is also a licensed clinical professional counselor who works part time as an adjunct psychology faculty at Bemidji State University.

———————

As a licensed clinical professional counselor and horse owner who specializes in EAP/EAL and human-animal interaction (HAI), my career involves diverse roles. After graduating with an undergraduate degree in applied psychology and a master's degree in counseling psychology from Bemidji State University, I have gone on to explore opportunities and work in clinical practice, teaching, and research. I also became certified through Eagala (Equine Assisted Growth and Learning Association) and opened a private practice, specializing in EAP. As a lifelong horse lover, I feel blessed to work in the field of EAP and AAI, helping people heal through this powerful work. I am also excited to be entering my second year of teaching as an adjunct psychology instructor at BSU, my alma mater.

My interest in HAI is rooted in my rural northern Minnesota upbringing on a ranch with horses, sheep, and a variety of other animals. Horses became a touchstone, connecting my soul to the natural rhythms of life. I spent hours studying and learning their unique language, riding, training, grooming, and caring for these magnificent animals. I eventually taught others (including my two sons) to ride and train. Time with horses brought me insight, confidence, and a sense of peace that planted the seed for eventually creating a private practice. For decades I have been using natural horsemanship training methods, incorporating nonviolent communication to instill trust, respect, and ultimately, a closer bond and working relationship with horses. These methodologies and practices cohesively apply to my work with both horses and humans.

My interest in the human-animal bond sparked the creation of Eagle Vista Ranch & Wellness Center (EVR), a for-profit, private practice which serves children to adults through EAP, personal development, and animal-assisted therapy. EVR also collaborates with BSU on HAI and AAI research projects, with an intent to increase awareness of the efficacy and process of these modalities. As a result, I have gone on to co-author various works and present nationally, and internationally as far away as Australia, on HAI research.

My schedule varies with the seasons; during summer months I spend early mornings doing chores and office work, then meet with clients for therapy sessions in the outdoor riding-arena or pasture into the late afternoon. During the school year I typically spend three mornings a week on campus (or online) teaching, followed by meeting with clients at Eagle Vista Ranch and processing clinical notes. In summer and fall we periodically contract with organizations and haul horses to off-site locations to provide equine-assisted services. Wintertime brings sub-zero temperatures to Bemidji, the "Icebox of America," hence, we offer therapy sessions in our indoor riding arena.

As a practitioner I face vexing challenges, perhaps most externally noticeable is that my office is both in my home and my barn, making it difficult to *leave work at the office*. To maintain healthy boundaries around my time and energy caring for both humans and animals, I have learned to delegate tasks to team members when feasible. Internal battles center upon the emotional fatigue called "compassion fatigue" that comes from being the support-arm for those who have suffered traumatic life-experiences.

Over the years I have developed a balance between struggles and rewards. I refill my emotional bucket by being with friends and family, riding horses, running, skiing, traveling, and other activities. The most rewarding parts of my job include harnessing the creative energies of our team members (*two-legged and four-legged*) to help transform lives through AAI, mentorship, teaching, and research. It also recharges and refuels me when clients gain insight and awareness through AAI. Mentoring and supervising interns and volunteers is also gratifying, and I am so pleased every time I hear from interns who embark upon graduate school and find stable employment in the field of AAI.

As a mental health professional and business owner annual income can vary anywhere from the $50,000 range to six figures, depending upon areas of specialization, the caseload of private practice clients, and any additional contracting or consulting. Teaching adds additional income, but personally my true currency is in the sharing of knowledge and experience with interested and engaged learners.

In response to the COVID-19 pandemic, our team recently created "Resilience & Recovery for Helping Professionals," a six-week online course (via Zoom) featuring EAL. This course addresses complex and delicate balances between caring for others vs. self-care in efforts to mitigate hazards of practice such as compassion fatigue, vicarious trauma, and burnout in the helping professions. We are also co-facilitating a six-week EAL group on Zoom with three other EAP/EAL professionals.

For those interested in investigating HAI work, I suggest taking particular steps, and as my grandfather used to say, "Do it *now*." Tour an animal-assisted facility; interview a mental health professional, equine specialist, animal specialist, or animal handler; and attend a network meeting, training, or conference (like Eagala) that features HAI programming. Finally, consider volunteering or doing an internship or practicum where animals are incorporated, for enriching experiences and unique perspectives as you navigate a career path in HAI.

52 Applying Theoretical Frameworks and Organizational Structures to Help Develop the Field of Animal-Assisted Interventions

The Questions We Must Ask and the Answers We Must Seek . . .

Katarina Felicia Lundgren

Katarina Felicia Lundgren is the Director of MiMer Centre—Equine-Human Education and Research and Centre, a nonprofit and research trust organization. She is also a nature-based trauma sensitive/informed mindfulness instructor who is currently training to become an expressive arts educator.

My interest in the field of animal-assisted interventions (AAI) is to increase quality of life for clients while guaranteeing the welfare of the animals involved. After managing a small unconventional equestrian center, I transitioned to offering equine-assisted psychotherapy and learning (EAP/L) to corporations, groups, and individuals. I also founded a non-profit organization, MiMer, a small equine-human research and education center, a trust that soon will support our field with funds for research and education. Today MiMer consists of a growing international network of dedicated researchers, educators, therapists, and others within the fields of animal science or human mental health, growth, and development. Together we explore and educate about the mechanisms in human-equine interaction, focusing on therapeutic interventions.

MiMer's goal is to establish treatment centers for trauma that conduct research on equines, their welfare, and equine-human interaction. We focus on therapy and learning situations from a scientific and model-independent perspective. It is greatly rewarding when participants become as fascinated by this work as we are—when they see the science beyond the set of tools they are given—and delve into the theoretical and experiential questions, becoming aware of their own individual, cultural, and scientific/educational biases. I started on this path wanting to offer EAP/L, but ended up seeking answers to some essential questions: Who is the horse? Why a horse? What is happening between a horse and a client in EAP/L? From there, the questions grew exponentially . . .

Today I spend my time engaged in research, education projects, international trainings, and educational events. I also dedicate time to develop MiMer as a collaborative network to further education, research, and treatment options in our field.

What initially set me on this career path were the first EAP/L trainings that I took in 2012 and my personal experiences as a recipient of equine-assisted trauma therapy (EATT). I attended these trainings knowing how effective equine-human interaction can be for human psychological, cognitive, and social development. The trainings confirmed this knowledge. But what they did not give were answers to my questions: Why is this work so powerful? What makes EAP/L have these profound effects on humans? What role does the horse play? What about the welfare of the horse? Full of questions, I enrolled in academic and non-academic courses to learn more about the cognition, behaviors, emotions, and social life of equines, equine-human interaction, and human cognition, psychology, and traumatology.

The challenges existing in our field include the lack of:

- Knowledge and research on equines and equine-human interaction
- Educational opportunities (preferably connected to universities) providing necessary theoretical knowledge and practical skills
- The availability of networks to help people build sustainable EAP/L businesses; supervisors, mentors, and partners; and specialized advanced educational opportunities
- Organizations to regulate the field (including ethical considerations), certify educational programs, connect researchers and providers, and facilitate networking opportunities
- Theoretical and contextual frameworks to better understand the mechanisms behind the interventions

Being part of a transdisciplinary movement where we look at AAT through multiple lenses—neurobiology, psychology, traumatology, sociology/social work, cognitive science, animal behavior and cognition, HAI, biology/zoology, ethology, anthrozoology, etc. helps us to better understand our interventions and to define our own field. The presence of animals makes for an extremely rich environment that provides an experiential situation brimming with possibilities, making AAT a powerful and multi-faceted approach full of potential. However, the transdisciplinary nature of the field may lead it to be misunderstood and misused in a way that can be detrimental to clients and animals. Best practice needs to be reached by deepening both theoretical and practical knowledge in our field, not by following old traditions and habits. Further scientific exploration of these mechanisms is needed to help us better understand our methods and our objectives.

Work in this field demands a great deal of research on the models you are interested in. Look for academic HAI programs. One must find a good network, engage in it, and find good collaborators, mentors, and supervisors. This field is still in its infancy and lacks structure and organizations with an overview. Contact someone who seems to share your professional values. Ask to join them, learn from them, and take trainings with them. Read the professional literature. This field is still in a phase where you must shape your own path. I wish you good luck! It is hard to find your way, but greatly rewarding when you do!

53 For the Love of Horses

Fay McCormack

Fay McCormack specialises in the field of addiction and has worked in an out-patient youth service while in the USA, and in residential and community-based drug and alcohol services in Australia. Her love of horses resulted in becoming a dual Eagala certified practitioner and establishing the first Equine-Assisted Therapy program within a Community Health Service in Australia. The program provides sessions for children, adolescents, women, men and groups experiencing a wide range of mental and psychosocial issues.

I have loved horses since I was a child. My father had a small property, and I was given a horse at age 10 to periodically muster the cattle. Monty was a chestnut Galloway with a blaze. He became a best friend, teacher and confidant. We went to Pony Club and Gymkhanas, competed in local shows and spent weekends exploring the countryside.

In terms of my education and early career path, I completed year 10, as was expected in my day, and worked in clerical jobs. Twenty years later, I decided to go to University after becoming a single mother of three children, much to my family's surprise. I completed a bachelor of arts with distinction achieving majors in psychology, welfare studies, sociology and geography at the University of Central Queensland. I worked in a variety of positions in Rockhampton and Moranbah before choosing to specialise in the field of addiction. In 2001, I became the first Australian to complete a master of arts in addiction counselling at the Hazelden Graduate School of Addiction Studies, Center City, Minnesota. I then worked in an out-patient youth treatment center in Stillwater, Minnesota. Since my return to Australia, I have worked in residential and community-based drug and alcohol services in Victoria.

While not having contact with horses since age 20, my love for them never dampened. After investigating two other models of Equine-Assisted Therapy and Equine-Assisted Learning, I chose the Eagala Model. Eagala necessitates "unlearning" many of one's professional skills as a mental health practitioner or as an equine specialist. The Eagala Model has a team approach, ground-based activities, is solution-oriented and sets global ethical standards promoting the physical and emotional safety of the horses and the clients (Eagala, 2015). I completed my Eagala training in Sydney in late 2011, and HAY (Horses Assisting You) began in early 2012. HAY is the only Equine-Assisted Therapy program within a Community Health Service in Australia.

Now in our ninth year, we have worked with a wide range of clients with various psychological, behavioural and environmental challenges including clients with drug and alcohol issues, women and children who have escaped family violence, children and adolescents in out-of-home care, adults and children who experienced the Black Saturday bushfires, individuals with mental health issues, and children on the autism spectrum. We also provide team building, leadership and personal development sessions.

A typical day at HAY starts at 8:30am and finishes at 5pm. Emails and messages are checked, and paperwork and supplies for the day are gathered before driving up to 45 minutes to a site for the day's sessions. Case notes are completed after each session, emails and messages are checked again, and phone calls (and lunch) are scheduled between sessions. My co-facilitator and I debrief after each session and prepare for our next session.

I have been extremely fortunate to have three certified Eagala practitioners with their own horses and properties within easy driving distance who have contracted to work for HAY. As a team, we have developed open and honest relationships based on mutual respect. These relational elements are essential as we check in with each other before sessions, work collaboratively during sessions and plan our clients' next session. The benefits of being in a team include: not having to have mental health qualifications and be an equine specialist; not having to have all the ideas and answers for every client or group; reduced isolation; and keeping everyone's ego in check. The team approach adds to the emotional and physical safety of the client and the horses.

In order to become competent in your chosen profession, you will need to deepen your theoretical knowledge and practice your skills for some years before venturing into Equine-Assisted Therapy. By doing this, the best interest of your client remains at the forefront. As with any profession, you always need to work within your scope of practice (Australian Counselling Association, 2016). Additional strengths and attributes needed to succeed include good time management and organisational abilities, and excellent communication skills.

During your time of exploration, find out who is practising Equine-assisted sessions in your area, attend their open days or ask to experience a session. Learn as much as you can about the animal-assisted therapy industry. Watch YouTube videos and explore relevant websites. Choose a model of Equine-Assisted Therapy that suits *your* values, your personality and the way you would like to work with horses.

Whichever model you choose, become involved with like-minded practitioners, attend networking meetings and volunteer as a way of broadening your knowledge. Be willing to continue to learn and to challenge yourself! I wish you all the best in your journey of discovery.

References

Australian Counselling Association. (2016). *Scope of practice for registered counsellors.* Newmarket, Queensland. https://www.theaca.net.au/documents/ACA%20Scope%20of%20 Practice%20for%20Registered%20Counsellors%202016.pdf

Eagala. (2015). *Fundamentals of the EAGALA model* (8th ed.). California, CA: Eagala.

54 Please Bear With Me— Working With My Canine Co-Therapist

Janus Moncur

Janus Moncur LCSW, CCTP, CHAIS, is a licensed clinical social worker, working on her PhD in social work. She specializes in trauma and canine-assisted therapy and is a certified clinical trauma professional (CCTP), compassion fatigue professional (CCFP), and, human animal intervention specialist (CHAIS). Janus volunteers as an instructor and handler with her own canine partners in disaster/crisis situations for National Crisis Response Canines.

Being raised in Inkster, Michigan, as an only child by a single mother, and then moving to Big Rapids, Michigan, at the age of 8 with Mom and my new stepdad, I was lucky to meet my best-friend, Heidi, that same year. Heidi, her family, and her home at the Circle W Ranch allowed me to become immersed into the amazing magic of animals. My mother astutely permitted me to spend as much time as possible with Heidi and the Ranch, and I am certain that my sanity and stability come from that escape. Learning responsibility and hard work that comes with caring for animals and receiving the rewards of love and unconditional acceptance is something I wish all children could experience in their lives. This experience guided the rest of my life and increased my love of animals.

My early college years included business school as I did not believe I could handle the science and math requirements involved in becoming a veterinarian. My career life was a corporate life, filled with brokerage firms, property management and real estate companies. I never felt happy or satisfied but rather, that I was chasing money. The real estate/mortgage crash of 2008 coupled with the medical emergency of my significant other (S.O.) required me to re-evaluate my whole life.

During my time as caregiver for my S.O., Denny, I witnessed the miracle of the power of puppy love, literally. I moved into Denny's home with my two old rescue dogs and proceeded to attempt to navigate the world of transplant medicine and being the girlfriend to a man with four teenage kids and an ex-wife. During the madness, the youngest daughter coaxed her father into buying a tiny Pomeranian puppy from a reputable breeder, so Jack was added to the mix.

I had a variety of dogs with me during the entire time Denny and I had known each other, but he was convinced he was allergic to dogs and never touched any of them. It was not that he did not like my dogs, but he had never bonded with a dog. The first night that Jack was brought home, he ignored his young mistress as she went off to bed and instead, sat at Denny's feet and demanded to be picked up. From that moment on, Denny and Jack became inseparable and it was apparent to all that Jack was now Daddy's dog.

Through that journey of relocating to Indianapolis for 14 months, from our sunny home in Florida, Jack was my partner. He was the only being that could wake the irritable sickly man and was the only being that could make him smile and laugh. I believe that without Jack, Denny's outcome could have been much different.

Shortly after the successful transplant, and with Jack's approval, another Pomeranian puppy came into our pack, Mack. Jack and Mack teamed up to become a powerhouse as we trained and became certified through Canine-Assisted Therapy, Inc. At the same time, I had returned to school to obtain my master of social work degree. It did not dawn on me until one of my professors, Dr. Janet Courtney, pointed out that I was already doing therapy work with the help of my dogs.

Today, I am a licensed clinical social worker in private practice and am known best for my work in trauma and work with my canine co-therapists. Today I work with a four-year-old keeshond named Pandora's Peter Bear. Bear's mother was rescued and gave birth to him the day after she was saved and now he works as my canine co-therapist after gaining his certificates. Most of my clients are adults who have suffered with addiction problems and/or trauma, although we have worked with children and adolescents as well. I conduct group therapy and work one-on-one with clients. My canine co-therapist and I travel to different facilities about 30 hours a week. I see clients in my private office and via teleconferencing. I love the positive energy that is ignited when clients see my canine partner. I get to hear greetings of "Bear! Bear! It's Bear! Hi, Bear!" Suddenly the prospect of going to group becomes happy anticipation. I am most rewarded when witnessing the wisdom of my canine partner as he hones in on clients who are struggling. The look of amazement and appreciation from the client and other group members is always heartwarming and revalidating as my partner sits with the struggling client.

My greatest challenge has been to help other health care providers and agencies embrace the "power of the pooch". Although the practice is more mainstream today, there is still so much unawareness and therefore, hesitancy by decision makers to allow canines into many facilities and centers. Yet, I feel this can be overcome with a great deal of patience and educating on the part of the practitioner. My advice about attempting to work in these facilities is to not take rejection personally for yourself or your dog(s). My most important piece of advice is to continue to learn and grow as a partner with your dog. Continue your education about the human/animal bond and continue to train and expose your partner to various situations that might be encountered. But most of all, become attuned to your canine's language, stress signals, and needs, just as you need to become aware of your own stress signals that transmit easily to your canine. Take care of each other, advocate for your partner, and do not take your partner for granted.

I am not sure that most people would have considered my 2008 as a positive situation, but it was for me. Being in the position to close my real estate business and take care of my favorite person, and the opportunities and life lessons that appeared because of all these events served as the catalyst for the truly amazing and happy life I live today.

55 Counselling With a Therapy Animal

Patricia Nitkin

Patricia Nitkin, PhD, CCC, is a clinical professor and the Clinic Director of the SFU Surrey Counselling Centre in the Master's program in counselling psychology at Simon Fraser University in British Columbia, Canada. She also runs a part-time private practice offering individual and group work with her therapy dog assistant George. Patricia offers relational and existential-humanistic therapies with the adjunctive approaches of Mindful Self Compassion, animal-assisted therapy and music therapy.

I named my companion-animal George Harrison after my favourite Beatle, because George is a remarkably present, peaceful, loving and deep rescue-dog. He accompanies me in my psychotherapy practice where I work with individuals, couples and families struggling with relational challenges, grief, trauma and/or mental-health issues. As many dogs do, George *reads* each person who enters the office and responds uniquely to the way they are *in that moment*. It marks the beginning of what will hopefully be a healing experience.

Early in my life and career, it became clear to me that companion-animals often provide extraordinary support to the humans in their world. I worked in palliative care and psychosocial-oncology, witnessing firsthand how patients, family members and staff relied on their companion-animals, speaking of them in profoundly grateful and loving ways. Many of them longed to be near their animal-companions and suffered when building or organizational regulations prohibited this. I experienced this myself through multiple painful losses. So after 20 years, I decided to pursue my Ph.D. in counselling psychology and study the human-animal bond (Nitkin & Buchanan, 2020).

In 2012 with the backing of research and some additional training, George joined me in his first session with a client who requested his presence. That was eight years ago, and George has been a partner in my counselling practice ever since. On a typical day George lays on the floor by the feet of the client or on the couch beside them during the session. He is on the couch strictly by the client's invitation and jumps down when either of them wishes. Some clients lay their heads on him as they weep. Others pet him rhythmically as they disclose painful life experiences, or they laugh when he yawns or snores. George gazes at them lovingly, at other times looks away knowingly, often falling asleep on their lap or by their feet. It is moving to witness, and clients share that his presence significantly contributes to a safe and healing environment.

George's interactions with clients offer relational exchanges that can be profoundly therapeutic and healing. However, incorporating George into my practice has required serious ethical and clinical consideration. Bringing another sentient being into the counselling experience is complex. What follows are some of the considerations I believe are critical to including a therapy animal (TA) in clinical counselling.

Clinical and Ethical Considerations

- It is essential that any TA be professionally trained for the work, and unfortunately, this training remains limited in availability. While we may adore them, our companion-animals may be unwelcome or dangerous to some. All clients must be informed of and given the choice ahead of time to have a TA's presence in session. As such, you may need additional space in your office where your TA can be comfortable and safe during sessions where they are not of benefit.
- It is essential that you include your TA in any and all legal and ethical considerations of your practice including professional liability insurance, client consent forms, rental contracts and building permits. Many office buildings only permit service-animals. If you share an office with other practitioners, they and their clients must be informed in case of allergies, fears or phobias.
- Psychotherapy is challenging work. Endeavouring to assist another person who is suffering and seeking your help requires skill, depth and full presence. With a TA, you now have another creature for which you are responsible. Will this distract you from your focus on the client?
- Counselling is emotionally charged and energetically dynamic. It's important to ensure that your TA is comfortable physically and emotionally during sessions. Are they overburdened by the energetic exchanges? I take George out for air after every second session and a run in an open space after each workday. Water, treats and food must be readily available, and the temperature in the room must consider their comfort as well as your clients' and your own.
- You likely love your TA and will watch for the way your clients treat them. What would you do if they held the animal so tightly that they yelped? How might this impact the therapeutic alliance? And how would you deal with your TA if they became frightened, upset or needy during a client session?
- As George gets older, both my clients and I are aware he won't live forever. Another impending loss can cause additional emotional suffering for a client, in particular those struggling to cope with grief.

- There is also the matter of touch. The majority of my clients welcome George's warm physical proximity. Your TA may want to be touched and given attention by clients; this can be rich therapeutic work, however, it may also be unsettling or too much of a focus in session. Additionally, clients who have experienced unwanted touch or sexual assault may experience a TA's bids for touch as unsafe.
- Finally, George and I became a popular duo for clients with dog phobias as well as those experiencing pet bereavement. As such I pursued further training in exposure therapy as well as companion-animal grief. Be prepared to expand your training to serve new presenting issues and needs in an ethical and clinically sound manner.

These are a few of the considerations I urge mental-health professionals to contemplate. I do so with the knowledge that the benefits of George's presence far outweigh any challenges I have faced. The richness of working with people who are struggling is an honour, and George's presence is a gift. Having a TA as a counselling-assistant, however, involves real emotional, legal and physical risks as well as a myriad of benefits and relational magic.

*Therapy animal: Currently the field of animal-assisted therapy is rapidly evolving and there is little to no standardization regarding the definition or certification of a therapy animal. I use this term with a descriptive stance.

Reference

Nitkin, P., & Buchanan, M. (2020). Relationships between people with cancer and their companion animals: What helps and hinders. *Anthrozoos, 33*(2), 243–259. https://doi.org/10.1080/08927936.2020.1719764

56 Forget Me Not Farm—A Haven for Children and Animals to Bond and Break the Cycle of Abuse

Carol M. Rathmann

Carol M. Rathmann is the Founder and Director of Forget Me Not Farm Children's Services since its inception in 1992. The farm offers animal assisted and horticultural therapeutic activities for child victims of abuse and neglect. The farm serves a variety of social service agencies that bring groups of children to the farm weekly for hour-long sessions. Carol is responsible for developing the farm's best practice model for animal assisted therapeutic interventions.

I have worked in the animal welfare industry since 1970. In 1991, while working at the local SPCA which held contract for animal control, I became interested in the human–animal bond when I discovered research connecting animal abuse to human violence.

As the shelter manager and coordinator of veterinary services I saw first-hand how people who were abusive to their animals were often aggressive to humans. It was at this time that California was in the process of legislating Animal Control Officers as mandated reporters of child abuse.

Attending workshops on the connection between child abuse and animal abuse, I began to educate myself about the cycle of violence and soon became obsessed with the need to break that cycle.

My first course associated with this field was through Harcum College in cooperation with The Devereux Foundation and the University of Pennsylvania School of Veterinary Medicine. The class was taught via cassette tapes and weekly teleconferencing. When I completed the class I received a Certificate of Achievement as a Specialist in Animal Assisted Activities and Therapy.

In 2000 I enrolled in a graduate program at Vermont College where I was able to design my own master of arts degree curriculum. My focus in that program was identifying the benefits of animal assisted therapy to children with attachment disorders. As a result of my studies, I began exploring the idea of teaching kindness toward animals to children who were victims of abuse and neglect—the antithesis of what they were witnessing at home.

This led to the development of Forget Me Not Farm. This farm is located on a 3-acre parcel behind the Humane Society of Sonoma County and is home to over 50 rescued farm animals and 2 acres of organic vegetable gardens. At the farm we offer animal assisted and horticultural therapeutic activities that provide a sanctuary for children, animals, and plants to interact, bond, learn, and heal. The farm is a place where children learn kindness, compassion, respect, empathy, and the makings of healthy relationships from new mentors they can trust, helping to break the cycle of abuse.

When I started this program I was a regular employee at the Humane Society, so I was able to enjoy a full-time salary as I built the animal assisted program. I incorporated the farm program into my regular work day and relied on trained volunteers to help. Attaching this program to an existing non-profit gave immediate credibility and made fundraising easier.

In 1992 our first group of children who had substantiated reports of abuse and neglect began their weekly visits to Forget Me Not Farm. The children came from a therapeutic preschool run by the Young Women's Christian Association (YWCA) of Sonoma County.

The first visit to Forget Me Not Farm can be intimidating for children who have not been around farm animals, but the use of farm animals in this program is intentional. Children from violent homes rarely experience gentle touch or empathy. The use of large, sturdy farm animals presents an opportunity for children to learn what it takes to develop a relationship with a living being without the use of force. In order to interact with the resident farm animals, the child(ren) often have some new behaviors to learn that include but are not limited to: impulse control, team work, and following directions.

The program was instantly popular with the referring agencies because they saw immediate improvement in the behavior of the children attending the farm program. Through word of mouth the program grew from six to 90 children per week. We currently serve over 350 at-risk children each year, and there is a waitlist for our services.

As the Founder and Director of Forget Me Not Farm, one of my greatest rewards is seeing previous clients returning to the animal shelter with lost or stray animals. As adults they are empathetic, kind caregivers to their own animals and to their human families. Several have returned to the farm as volunteers, and some have become animal foster parents at the local shelter. One graduate of the program was recently hired to work at the farm.

Developing a program like Forget Me Not Farm has been a challenge because animal welfare and animal control agencies often focus on pet adoptions and licensing and their humane education often centers around spay/neuter. The typical animal assisted therapy program in animal shelters involves volunteers visiting nursing homes, hospitals, schools and libraries. The theory that teaching at-risk youth to be kind to animals will eventually reduce animal abuse and relinquishment is not yet widely understood or accepted.

Animal assisted therapy is not yet recognized as a therapeutic discipline and therefore raises a lot of questions about what it is and who can provide it. When I started this work there were very few education options and online learning was not readily available. Today there are more options. There is a Humane Animal Bond Certification program offered online by the North American Veterinary Community (NAVC) and the Human Animal Bond Research Institute (HABRI) as well as other online programs.

For those thinking about offering large animal AAI, I would suggest the following:

Identify local organizations with existing facilities and staff who are already caring for farm animals. This may be a large animal rescue organization or your local animal shelter or humane society. Volunteer your time and see if it would be feasible to create a program onsite.

Large animal programs can be expensive. They require acreage, barns, feed, veterinary care, and someone to be onsite every day. Partnering with an existing agency will reduce or eliminate these costs and allow you time to develop a program and a fundraising strategy while you are gaining experience and making community connections.

57 Integrating Human–Animal Interactions and Psychology

Research and Service

Yahaira Segarra

Yahaira Segarra, PhD, is the Subdirector of the master's program of counseling psychology at Albizu University in Puerto Rico. She offers continuing education and teaches a graduate course on human-animal interactions (HAI) and animal-assisted interventions (AAI). Yahaira has trained on animal-assisted interventions in the United States and Colombia. She has two registered therapy dogs that accompany her during animal-assisted psychotherapy (AAP) sessions.

I grew up surrounded by cats, dogs, rabbits, roosters, and fish, but the most influential for me were dogs. When I went to college to study psychology, I questioned if there were psychologists interested in our relationships with companion animals, and if any have wondered about the possible benefits of integrating animals in their work. For me this was not mere curiosity, but a topic worth studying. I started researching and I was surprised to find that, in fact, there was work on this topic. I found Dr. Boris Levinson's pet-oriented child psychotherapy book and the Delta Society Organization's work (now known as Pet Partners) and felt that I had a found a place where I belonged. I felt that I too could contribute to the study of the human-animal bond, and, ideally, could practice AAP.

I finished my undergraduate degree, completed a master's degree in mental health counseling and started a PhD program in counseling psychology. When time came to propose my dissertation project, I knew I wanted it to be about HAI. This was back in 2009, and in Puerto Rico (PR) AAI and the human-animal bond were topics scarcely studied. Finding a mentor was also challenging, since most professors saw HAI work as trivial. I remember one even telling me that it was a fad. Finally, I found a mentor; she was not an animal lover, but she believed in me as a student and was willing to take the risk. I was able to complete my PhD with a dissertation about general well-being and pet attachment in older adults living in the western region of PR and had the opportunity to present my work at the International Association of Anthrozoology (ISAZ) Conference in 2012.

In the meantime, I met a local group dedicated to animal-assisted activities (AAA) called Puerto Rico Therapy Dogs. They are part of the Alliance of Therapy Dogs, Inc. In 2012, I registered my first therapy dog with them and started doing volunteer work in hospitals, schools, and universities. Nothing made me happier that watching people interact with my golden retriever Astro. Later, my husband rescued a stray dog that we named Pecas that also became registered, and as a family we got involved in AAA, making it a part of our lives.

One of the most rewarding HAI experiences for me was collaborating with a non-profit called Surf 4 DEM that works with children and youth with neurodevelopmental disorders through adapted surfing. Every other weekend we would take the dogs to the beach to interact with their participants while they waited for their turn to surf. Together with the dogs, we helped these children with eye contact, social interaction, and sensory stimulation. Doing those visits, watching the progress that the surf therapists made with the kids and the sense of community that the families of those participants built was captivating.

It was during this time that I opened my private practice, including AAP as a complementary modality I used primarily with teenagers. It was helpful having the dogs in office, facilitating rapport building and making it easier for clients to open up, engage, and adhere to treatment. I witnessed how the dogs were key in assisting my clients in achieving their treatment goals. Locally I was nicknamed "*la doctora de los perros*" (the doctor with dogs).

Furthermore, I started teaching undergraduate and graduate level courses. At the University of Puerto Rico, Mayaguez Campus, I also created the first *De-stress Day*. This initiative was created to help college students relax on the days before their finals by spending time with visiting therapy dogs. Given its success, a group of students, guided by the campus' wellness office, founded a program called Puppy RUM that has continued AAA and animal welfare initiatives.

Moreover, to advance my knowledge in the area, I took several AAI trainings (e.g., Animal-Assisted Therapy Programs of Colorado, Corpoalegría in Colombia, and the Institute of Human-Animal Connection at the University of Denver). As a result, I teach graduate counseling psychology students, support students who are pursuing this research area, and offer the first elective course about HAI and AAI at Albizu University. I also teach about HAI to professionals through continuing education workshops.

What I would suggest somebody considering integrating HAI in his or her work:

- Search for high quality research done in their specific area of interest
- Realize that you will need to find further HAI specific training
- When considering doing AAI work, remember that it is not only about humans' welfare, but also about the non-human animals

- Attend an ISAZ, International Association of Human-Animal Interaction Organizations (IAHAIAO), or Animals on the Mind Conference
- Interview local professionals or organizations doing HAI work
- Shadow those doing HAI work
- Network with others interested in the field

58 The Art and Science of Equine Facilitated Psychotherapy

Marilyn Sokolof

Marilyn Sokolof, PhD, is a licensed psychologist, PATH Intl Equine Special-ist in Mental Health and Learning, and a PATH therapeutic riding instruc-tor. She is Developer/Director of Unbridled Therapy, a training program for professionals interested in equine facilitated psychotherapy (EFP); Clini-cal Director of HorseMpower, Inc., and faculty/evaluator for the PATH ESMHL Workshop/Skills Test. She recently retired as Director of Equine Psychotherapy at a residential addictions treatment center.

––––––––––

As a practicing psychologist for 40+ years, the "is-it-art or is-it-science" issue has remained a dogged question. The obvious answer is the field requires both approaches: the science that expands our understanding of, and confidence in, what we do, and the art that allows for the spontaneity and creativity that is part of our daily practice. Add in horses, and the art/science issue becomes even more important in determining what the best practices are for a relatively young industry and profession. As a practitioner of EFP for 20+ years, I offer my story in hopes that it can provide some insight for the field.

The science part of my story was primary as a graduate student. While hindsight has shown me the importance of biology, research, and mathemat-ics, at the time it felt mostly irrelevant. I wanted to HELP people. For the ensuing years, the art of providing psychotherapy was a rich experience, and yes I did HELP people. And, as the years marched on, the wide-ranging scientific discoveries did in fact help clarify best practices and assist me in the office.

Horses have been a magnificent part of my life from childhood. I love the sensual aspects—the way they smell, their physical presence—and am amused (and sometimes frustrated!) by their personalities. The experience of riding brings me true joy. The barn is a place for healthy physical challenge, emotional comfort, and true mindfulness. It has served as a great antidote for the many hours in the office spent witnessing so much pain.

It finally dawned on me that what horses do for me could be offered to my clients. Thirty years ago, setting up an EFP practice was more art than science. There were few resources. I was fortunate enough to find a small group of people (through North American Riding for the Handicapped Association [NARHA], now Professional Association for Therapeutic Horsemanship [PATH Intl]) but there was little science to aid in either best clinical or business practice. For those of you wanting to enter into in this field, the body of knowledge is growing exponentially, and I encourage you to examine it for opportunities and assistance. Modern technology affords you the ability to search for them easily.

In addition to providing EFP as a private practice and as Clinical Director of HorseMpower, Inc. (an EFP program in Gainesville, Fla.), I also developed and directed an EFP program at a residential treatment center for clients struggling with addiction and co-occurring disorders. Throughout my career, I have been privileged to be present for the exquisite interactions between horses and clients that allows for so much healing and self-discovery.

Retired now from direct service, I have focused my experience and knowledge into teaching others. I developed a training/consultation program "Unbridled Therapy" for both mental health as well as equine professionals. I am faculty for the PATH Intl workshop providing certification as an Equine Specialist in Mental Health and Learning. I am also a proud member of the Executive Committee for the organization Federation for Horses in Education and Therapy International (HETI), discovering people from all over the world who are engaged in equine-assisted interventions.

My advice for those of you interested in providing EFP:

- Be prepared for important revelations, emotional intensity, and rapid transformations—that is the power of this work. The moments in the barn are complex. Be prepared cognitively, but also emotionally. Work with populations with which you are already experienced. Allow for the "art" of witnessing those moments between client and horse. Be supportive, but do not interfere. Provide structure, but be flexible.
- Of primary importance is consideration of your equine partner. Know both the art and science of good horse care, physical and emotional. Give your horse a voice, and listen carefully to it, for everyone's sake (client, horse, and yourself). Do not disrespect your equine partner (or any animal) by defining them as "bombproof", "would never hurt you", etc.—denying their "animalness" denies them the right to have their basic instincts and behavior that comes from those instincts. Allow them to inform you and your clients.
- Be scrupulous about complying with safety standards, both physical and emotional.
- Be clear if this is a profession from which you expect to make income; learn about best business practices, follow guidelines, know your professional requirements, and don't skimp on them.
- Be a member of equine-assisted intervention professional organizations. Not only will you have access to the ever-growing body of resources

(programming, business, research, etc.), you will find support from like-minded individuals. Being on working committees for my entire EFP career has been educational and rewarding in many ways. And, I'm happy to give back to an industry that has done so much for me.

- Learn by attending workshops, reading material, and conversing with others—both "experts" as well as "newbies", the latter a hotbed of thinking outside the box.
- The science is important; read/study/search out as much information as you can. Your personal competencies are not only an ethical demand in working with clients; they will provide a foundation for those complex moments in the barn.
- Attend to your own mental health.

Mostly, I want to encourage. Follow your interest and passion; trust your instincts; seek doors that are open; believe in this process and all it has to offer.

59 Animal Assisted Play Therapy

Risë VanFleet

Risë VanFleet, PhD, RPT-S, CDBC, is a licensed psychologist, registered play therapist-supervisor, and certified dog behavior consultant. She is the President of the Family Enhancement and Play Therapy Center in Boiling Springs, Pennsylvania, and is a co-creator of the International Institute for Animal Assisted Play Therapy® (AAPT) which provides training and competence-based certification for professionals throughout the world.

I began preparing for new roles in Human-Animal Interaction (HAI) long before I knew that was where I was heading. Forty years ago, while serving as a live-in houseparent in a community mental health residential program when completing my master's degree, I did my first intervention when one of the residents wanted to set up a fish tank. Later, even though my doctoral focus was on working with children and families, I took courses in ethology and read a great deal about animal behavior simply out of interest. During the first decades of my career, while conducting therapy with children and families in private practice (as a family psychologist and play therapist), setting up a new family program in a hospital, serving as clinical director of a large community mental health center, working with mid-sized manufacturing companies to establish self-managed work teams, and traveling throughout the world conducting play therapy trainings for mental health professionals, I continued my "pleasure reading" of everything I could find—fiction and nonfiction—about dogs and horses. I also took numerous trips to Alaska to photograph Alaskan brown bears in the wild, where I learned more about applied ethology, animal behavior, and bear body language—an important thing to know if you are walking in the woods on bear paths or hiking along salmon streams and can bump into bears at any time! Even so, I had no plans to become involved in HAI, mostly because I was unaware of anyone doing this type of work.

My big shift to systematic HAI work occurred after nearly three decades in the mental health field. I was working with a foster child who had experienced horrific abuse, some questionable foster placements, and two failed adoptions. He did well with play therapy and Filial Therapy (a form of family therapy) with his foster mother, but I knew he still had remaining dilemmas that were difficult for him to work through. I did something I now tell others not to do—I took my very sociable, playful, and well-trained dog, Kirrie, to work with me. I held a session which worked exceptionally well. After this session, however, I realized I had much more to learn. All my prior reading alerted me to my need to develop more competencies. I then attended many animal behavior/training workshops. I volunteered my behavior consultation skills with local dog rescues—one of the best things I did to develop my hands-on skills and apply what I was learning. Eventually I became a certified dog behavior consultant, and I still conduct behavior consults with people and their dogs. Of greatest importance, I have used what I learned to co-develop the field of Animal Assisted Play Therapy® (AAPT) alongside mental health professional and equine behaviorist Tracie Faa-Thompson of the UK.

AAPT involves the integration of several fields, including psychotherapy, animal behavior, ethology, play therapy, and animal welfare. We operate from a set of principles that preserve the animal's well-being as well as that of the client. AAPT is appropriate for all ages and can be done with individuals, families, and groups. Practitioners develop many competencies to incorporate into their therapy work, including reading animal body language fluently, using animal-friendly positive training, building strong and reciprocal therapist-animal relationships, and involving animals in novel ways so they always have choices and enjoyable experiences.

My AAPT work has included a part-time private practice in which I conduct AAPT *pro bono*, as well as working full-time teaching professionals about AAPT, animal behavior, and more. We developed an independent certification program with rigorous requirements based on demonstrated competencies (see www.iiaapt.org). This program is active throughout the world, and there are certified AAPT professionals involving many species in their work, all following the relationship and animal well-being principles at the heart of all we do. My work also entails supervision, writing, course development, teaching course instructors, and organizational development to support and sustain those involved. It's immensely rewarding. The primary challenges are reaching the many people in our field who remain unaware of animals' perceptions and experiences in AAI, and helping them recognize and advocate for their animals when they are stressed.

Is There a Personality Type That's Better Suited to AAPT Work?

I will answer this from both human and animal points of view. For humans, I would say there is not. One must be able to split one's attention, read body language fluently, think proactively from the animal's point of view, and simultaneously conduct psychotherapy sessions effectively. That's a lot, but it can be learned by anyone who is motivated. It takes hard work, but it's well worth it in terms of the relationships one can develop with animals and clients. I think there's room in the HAI field for nearly everyone!

For animals, it is commonly thought that quiet, docile, obedient animals are the best therapy animals. I disagree! While this is likely true for visitation programs, in our AAPT work, we work with a wide range of animal personalities. Our way of doing so differs, though. Instead of expecting the animals to fit into the types of interventions clients need, we engage the animals in work that suits their personalities, energy levels, and interests. We use a goodness-of-fit model in which we select interventions based on (a) the client goals, (b) the animal's personality and interests, (c) the therapist's skills, and (d) the environment at the time. This works beautifully and allows us to involve many different animal personalities.

This is a most rewarding field, but it does take dedication and supervised experience to do well. The good news is that it is so fascinating to learn!

60 Create Your Herd
Developing a Career Through Lived Experiences

Aviva Vincent

Aviva Vincent, PhD, is a graduate of Case Western Reserve University, Mandel School of Social Welfare in veterinary social work. She is the Director of Program Quality at Fieldstone Farm Therapeutic Riding Center in Chagrin Falls, Ohio. She is also an instructor at Case Western Reserve University and teaches at the University of Tennessee in the Veterinary Social Work Certificate Program. Aviva is the Founder and a co-chair of the human-animal interactions workgroup with National Association of Social Workers, Ohio chapter.

It was my early childhood experiences with animals that attributed to my professional career trajectory. I grew up in a home working through a contemptuous divorce; in memories, at the barn was where I felt safe. Horses taught me empathy and compassion. They taught me that falling off, though painful, was an opportunity to get back on; they brought out my confidence and taught me trust.

Horses remain a central structure of my self-care. Through my master's program, I created the first equine social work field placement at Ebony Horsewomen Inc. in Hartford, Connecticut. This inner-city, therapeutic riding center was, and still is, a haven for youth from the community to learn horsemanship and engage in animal husbandry and gardening.

At EHI, I met a young man who had a temper that required time to quell. One day, he came to the farm from school in a terrible mood; his energy was emanating from his being. In silence, I followed him to the barn. I watched him as he walked up to the stall door and flung it open. The horse spun around so fast and feigned to kick him—but didn't. I saw the boy take stock of how close he had come to getting kicked. He stepped back, took a deep breath, and lowered his shoulders. Then he stepped back up to the open stall door and extended his hand. The horse lowered his head and allowed the young man to put his halter on. Together, they walked off.

The horse had mirrored his behavior and showed him that he needed to step back and breathe. *That* is the beauty of what horses teach us. In that moment, I also saw my child-self in that young man. I saw the hurt, unregulated young child who was looking for safety, comfort, and love. He found it in a horse, as did I. Being at EHI was a pivotal experience in my education and career trajectory; just as I had created my field placement, I could also create a career that merges social work practice and animals.

There is no singular path to working in human-animal interaction (HAI). My path to Veterinary Social Work was circuitous and came to fruition through volunteerism, internships, employment, networking, and mentorship. I credit dynamic mentors and my perseverance to ask questions, pursue education, and read copious amounts of literature.

My career path began with earning an undergraduate degree at the University of Massachusetts Amherst, then a master's in social work at the University of Connecticut, and my doctorate from Case Western Reserve University. To complement my degrees, I completed the Veterinary Social Work certificate program from the University of Tennessee, attended *Spit Camp* at the Institute for Interdisciplinary Salivary Bioscience at University of California at Irvine, participated in the inaugural fellowship at Animals & Society at University of Illinois, Urbana-Champaign, and completed my Professional Association of Therapeutic Horsemanship (PATH Intl) certified therapeutic riding instructor certification.

In my current position, I am privileged to "wear multiple hats" allowing me to stay emerged in multiple areas of HAI. In my primary position, I am the Director of Program Quality at Fieldstone Farm Therapeutic Riding Center in Chagrin Falls, Ohio. My responsibility is to ensure that our team provides the highest quality programming and services to every person who walks through the door. We do this by ensuring all instructors receive PATH Intl training and certification, creating a strong team environment where we learn and support each other, and engage in research to understand the impact of our programming.

I serve as adjunct faculty at Case Western Reserve University and University of Tennessee Veterinary Social Work certificate program (VSW-CP). Additionally, I am the co-owner of Healing Paws LLC, a Veterinary Social Work provider of education, resources, and support to Northeast Ohio.

If this sounds like the career path for you, here are some tips and tricks to get involved:

- Sign up for newsletters: Human Animal Bond Research Institute, Animals & Society, Veterinary Social Work.
- Join professional associations: American Psychological Association Human Animal Interaction Section, International Association of Veterinary Social Work, International Association of Anthrozoology, PATH Intl, EAGALA, National Association of Social Workers.

- Read journal articles. Using scholar.google.com, read peer-reviewed and alternative publications. A great resource for accessing articles and following authors is ResearchGate.net.

  - If you enjoy someone's writing, research, work in the community, connect with them! Send an email and ask them for tea/coffee, for an interview, or to be a mentor.

- Attend conferences, events, and workshops: Veterinary Social Work Summit, International Association of Anthrozoology, Animals on the Mind at Denver University, American Psychological Association.
- Education is an investment. Think ahead to where the field is going and what certifications, degrees, or learning may be helpful as you pursue your career.
- Seek and utilize mentors. Mentors are our champions, our confidants, and our advocates. In an emergent field, they are our network of support.
- Trust your curiosities and desires. Your career path may be non-traditional, or it may not fit neatly into a box—that is ok! Be persistent—create the career that will make you happy.

61 Canines, Equines, and Social Work

Heather White

Heather White, LMSW, is the owner of AIM HAI, LLC, an animal-assisted interactions consulting company. She is a professional dog trainer and mental health professional and was the Director of Programs and Training and an executive trainer at The Good Dog Foundation for several years. Heather holds a certificate in Animals and Human Health and Equine-Assisted Mental Health through the University of Denver's Institute for Human Animal Connection, a certificate in Treating Animal Abuse through Arizona State University, and a certificate in Veterinary Social Work through the University of Tennessee.

I've been an animal lover for as long as I can remember; little did I know this childhood love would grow into my current professional journey. I began a career in the field of human–animal interactions first as a professional dog trainer, followed by studies in Social Work. Social Work offered me the ability to combine my interests in social justice, equality, and of course, human–animal interactions. I was afforded the opportunity to advance my skills in both dog training and human–animal interactions in my work at a therapy dog organization while completing my master's degree in social work through Hunter College. During that time, I also completed the Animals and Human Health Certificate program through the University of Denver's Institute for Human Animal Connection, a thorough and well-developed foundation program. From there, I completed a program through Arizona State University, becoming familiar with the AniCare and AniCare Child models of working with those who have abused animals. Each opportunity for learning offered reinforcement and motivation for me that I had found a field that matched my interests and values.

My next step was completing the University of Tennessee's Veterinary Social Work (UT VSW) certificate program. This training pertains to multiple aspects of human–animal interactions, including Animal-Assisted Interactions, the link between human and animal violence, mediation and managing conflict, and compassion fatigue involved in human–animal interactions. UT's VSW program also focuses on animal-related grief and bereavement. It was during this coursework, that I began working at a local equestrian center focused on therapeutic riding and ground-based activities and was introduced to the myriad of methods, training, husbandry, and considerations involved in working with equines in a therapeutic capacity.

After completing my coursework in the VSW program, I came across the University of Denver's Equine-Assisted Mental Health Practitioner Program (EAMH). In this program, I gained a deeper understanding of equine ethology, animal welfare, the importance of trauma-informed care, professional competencies, and a greater picture of the field of professional mental health practice incorporating equines. I appreciated the carefully curated content and delivery focused on interpersonal awareness alongside ethological awareness. I also became involved with several other equine-assisted certifications and trainings and while I enjoyed many of them, the university-based programs have been the most beneficial educational experiences for me. It was in the EAMH program that the mental health practitioner aspect came full circle for me and re-engaged my desire to pursue additional education and experience in psychotherapy and Social Work.

In working towards my doctorate in social work and furthering my own knowledge base, I offer consultation and professional educational services to agencies, organizations, and individuals in the health and human services professions who are looking to incorporate human-animal interactions programming. The focus of these programs is always on mutually beneficial outcomes for the humans as well as the animals involved.

The best and most rewarding aspect of the jobs I have had is that no two days are ever the same. It's wonderful to have the opportunity to engage in interactions that are beneficial for all involved. It's also a great benefit that often times working with animals brings us outside of traditional work environments to a much more expansive outdoors work environment.

When it comes to workload and work/life balance, my workdays tend to be longer and involve non-traditional hours. Weekends easily become workdays, which feed into work weeks and before I know it, I've worked 20 days straight without a day away. You can definitely take this type of work home with you, planning ahead for tomorrow, emailing or texting with coworkers during off-hours, etc. I have worked remotely during vacations, and many nights on a laptop in an airport, hotel, or conference. An incredibly important aspect of any healthy work-life balance is to make sure to make time for yourself—something with which I still struggle. Finding an employer who understands a healthy work-life balance and follows it themselves is essential.

Other advice I would offer is to go to HAI related conferences and join networking groups to learn more and get involved. It's important to continue the journey of learning, not solely within one organization, but understanding human-animal interactions on a global scale.

As the field grows, there continues to be a well-defined separation between animal-assisted activities vs. psychotherapy practice incorporating animals. A correlating challenge is establishing competency standards for individuals involved in the field, guided by the ethics, education, profession, licensure, etc. of the specific discipline.

The field of human–animal interactions continues to expand at a rapid pace with professional roles within psychology, physiology, and education beginning to become more well-defined and organized. There is room for professionals from all lines of education and training to be involved in HAI work. It has truly been a pleasure to work within this growing field and meeting so many truly talented, educated, experienced people along the way. If it weren't for these individuals with immense vision, the field would not be what it is today. As long as humans and animals walk this world together, we will continue to evolve and grow in countless ways—we're interconnected.

Index

For Product Safety Concerns and Information please contact our EU
representative GPSR@taylorandfrancis.com
Taylor & Francis Verlag GmbH, Kaufingerstraße 24, 80331 München, Germany

www.ingramcontent.com/pod-product-compliance
Lightning Source LLC
Chambersburg PA
CBHW071414290326
41932CB00047B/2856